Colour Handbook of

OCCUPATIONAL DERMATOLOGY

John SC English
MB, FRCP
Consultant Dermatologist
Queen's Medical Centre
University Hospital
Nottingham, UK

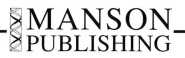
MANSON PUBLISHING

Copyright © 1998 Manson Publishing Ltd
ISBN 1-874545-58-8 (Cased edition)
ISBN 1-874545-91-X (Softcover edition)

A CIP catalogue record for this book is available from the British Library.

For full details of all Manson Publishing Ltd titles please write to
Manson Publishing Ltd, 73 Corringham Road, London NW11 7DL, UK.

Project Management: John Ormiston
Colour reproduction: Tenon & Polert, Hong Kong
Printed by: Grafos SA, Barcelona, Spain

CONTENTS

Contributors   iv
Foreword   v
Preface   vi
Acknowledgements   vi

Chapter One
Introduction to Occupational Skin Disease   1
John SC English

Chapter Two
Irritant Contact Dermatitis   11
Chee Leok Goh

Chapter Three
**Allergic Contact Dermatitis: Immunological Aspects and Common
Occupational Causes**   31
Neils K Veien

Chapter Four
**Occupational Skin Disorders Associated with
Sun or Artificial Light Exposure**   53
James Ferguson

Chapter Five
Miscellaneous Occupational Dermatoses   63
Michael H Beck and John SC English

Chapter Six
Differential Diagnosis of Hand Eczema   81
Henke B van der Walle

Chapter Seven
Occupational Dermatitis due to Plants and Woods   103
Christopher R Lovell

Chapter Eight
Occupational Acne   121
Craig Omohundro and James S Taylor

Chapter Nine
Occupational Skin Cancer   135
Rosemary Nixon

Chapter Ten
Pigmentary Changes Related to Occupation   147
David J Gawkrodger

Chapter Eleven
Occupational Connective Tissue Disorders   159
Volker Ziegler

Chapter Twelve
Occupational Skin Infections   169
John T Lear and John SC English

Index   182

CONTRIBUTORS

Michael H Beck
Consultant Dermatologist
The Skin Hospital
Manchester, England

John SC English
Consultant Dermatologist
Department of Dermatology
Queen's Medical Centre
University Hospital
Nottingham, England

James Ferguson
Consultant Dermatologist
Department of Photobiology
Ninewells Hospital
Dundee, Scotland

David J Gawkrodger
Consultant Dermatologist and
Honorary Clinical Lecturer in
Dermatology
Department of Medicine
University of Sheffield and Royal
Hallamshire Hospital
Sheffield, England

Chee Leok Goh
Clinical Associated Professor and
Medical Director
National Skin Centre
Singapore

John T Lear
Resident
North Staffordshire NHS Trust
Stoke-on-Trent, England

Christopher R Lovell
Consultant Dermatologist
Royal United Hospital
Bath, England

Rosemary Nixon
Dermatologist
206 Albert St
East Melbourne, Australia

Craig Omohundro
Dermatologist
Section of Industrial Dermatology
Cleveland Clinical Foundation
Cleveland
Ohio, United States of America

James S Taylor
Chairman
Section of Industrial Dermatology
Cleveland Clinical Foundation
Cleveland
Ohio, United States of America

Neils K Veien
Director
The Dermatology Clinic
Aalborg, Denmark

Henke B van der Walle
Director
Centrum Arbeidsdermatologie
Arnhem, The Netherlands

Volker Ziegler
Formerly Professor, Leipzig University
Skin Clinic
Bunde, Germany

FOREWORD

Occupational dermatoses are rivalled only by musculoskeletal disorders as the most common form of occupationally induced disease. Yet their diagnosis is still commonly missed altogether and, even when suspected, these dermatoses remain widely underinvestigated. There is, therefore, a pressing need for greater awareness among all those who may be presented with occupational skin disorders, including paramedics, safety representatives and nurses, as well as family physicians, dermatologists and occupational physicians.

General textbooks and atlases of dermatology are of only limited help in this respect, since the space that can be devoted to occupational dermatoses in these is usually only small. This exceptionally well-illustrated handbook is to be welcomed greatly, as it both encourages clinical suspicion and then enables this to be transformed into a provisional diagnosis, so that the appropriate investigations can be carried out. Helpful guidance is also given as to the subsequent management of such cases.

With this book at hand, the detection rate of occupational skin disorders cannot fail to be increased, as well as confidence instilled in the physician as to how to proceed to the investigation and management of such disorders.

I congratulate Dr English on the compilation of this handbook, and commend it to all those charged with the management of this common, but still widely underinvestigated, group of skin diseases.

Richard JG Rycroft
St John's Institute of Dermatology
St Thomas's Hospital
London

PREFACE

Occupational skin diseases are very common. Unfortunately, doctors, nurses, paramedics and safety officers receive very little training in this speciality. *Colour Handbook of Occupational Dermatology* is designed to make up this deficiency.

The main purpose of this colour handbook is to help those involved in occupational medicine and dermatology to diagnose occupational skin diseases; it complements textbooks on occupational diseases.

Most work-related skin disease is dermatitis and so other occupational skin problems are often forgotten. During the preparation of this book, I realised that a particularly unusual and unresponsive case of acne I was treating was chloracne brought about by polychlorinated biphenyls. If I had not read the chapter on chloracne the correct diagnosis probably would not have occurred to me. This book provides invaluable help to understand the causes, diagnosis, and management of occupational skin diseases.

John SC English
Queen's Medical Centre
Nottingham

ACKNOWLEDGEMENTS

I thank all my colleagues with whom I have worked over the years, especially Drs Etain Cronin, Richard Rycroft and Ian White at the Contact Clinic, St John's Hospital for Diseases of the Skin, London. I am most grateful to Stuart Robertson of the Institute of Dermatology, London, for an education on medical photography and for the use of several pictures in this book, and to Dr David Fitzgerald for the translation of Chapter 11 from German into English. Naturally, without the contributors this book would not have been possible and so to them, many thanks.

John SC English
Queen's Medical Centre
Nottingham

CHAPTER ONE

INTRODUCTION TO OCCUPATIONAL SKIN DISEASE

John SC English

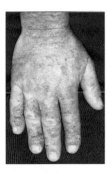

Contact dermatitis is common and often has a poor prognosis.

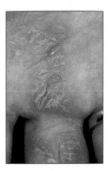

Psoriasis and other non-eczematous skin diseases can be aggravated by work.

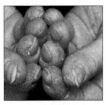

Irritants, allergens, and infection can all cause contact dermatitis.

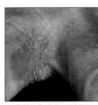

The correct final diagnosis cannot always be determined from the pattern of the dermatitis.

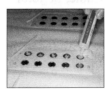

Bimodal distribution of age when contact dermatitis develops.

Patch testing is essential to elucidate the cause(s) of contact dermatitis.

PREVALENCE

Dermatitis is a common condition which probably affects from 15 to 20% of the UK population; many of these will have atopic dermatitis. However there are very few population-based studies specifically looking at the prevalence of hand dermatitis, especially occupational (*Table 1*).

Table 1. The prevalence of dermatitis from seven studies performed within the past 30 years.

Location	Site	Prevalence (%)
Faeroe Islands	All sites	1.7
Southern Sweden	Hands	0.6
Inner London	All sites	6.1
USA	All sites	4.7
USA	Hands	0.5
Netherlands	Hands and arms	6.2
Sweden	Hands	11.8

FREQUENCY

The majority of occupational dermatoses consist of contact dermatitis (*Table 2*). Accurate figures for the frequency of occupational contact dermatitis in the general population is not known – some authorities estimate the frequency as approximately 10/10 000/year (*Table 3*). Most governmental statistics are probably underestimates due to under-diagnosis or under-reporting. However, several initiatives world-wide are being undertaken to obtain more accurate figures. There are many published surveys looking at the prevalence of contact dermatitis in factories where there have been dermatitis problems. These are usually isolated epidemics. In the Stoke-on-Trent pottery industry, however, certain wet-work jobs such as lithography have an approximate 10% prevalence of low grade contact dermatitis of the hands. In a Swedish survey, high figures of 21.3%, were found for hand dermatitis in cleaners, compared with other occupations of approximately 11%. The prevalence of hand dermatitis in women was twice as high as for men.

Traditionally, occupational skin diseases have been the most prevalent of all the occupational health problems, however musculoskeletal problems are now much more common (*Table 4*).

Table 2. The UK surveillance reporting scheme (EPI-DERM) for occupational skin disease 1993–1995 by dermatologists and occupational physicians.

Diagnosis	Dermatologists (%)	Occupational physicians (%)
Contact dermatitis	79.8	76.7
Contact urticaria	3.0	3.7
Infective	1.6	8.4
Neoplasia	13.2	0.4
Other	4.6	11.5

Table 3. Occupations with the highest risk rate (/10 000/year) using labour force survey data as the denominator and contact dermatitis and urticaria from the UK EPI-DERM survey.

Dermatologists	Rate (/10 000/year)	Occupational physicians	Rate (/10 000/year)
Hairdressers	10.9	Chemical workers	20.7
Printers	7.1	Biological scientists	6.9
Foundry workers	6.2	Machine tool operators	6.8
Beauticians	5.1	Electroplaters	6.2
Machine tool operators	4.9	Vehicle assemblers	4.5

Table 4. Work-related health problems as reported by UK occupational physicians during 1996.

Problem	Percentage
Musculoskeletal	45.3
Dermatological	23.4
Respiratory	9.2
Hearing loss	8.7
Other	13.9

There is no doubt that occupational contact dermatitis is also very costly to society as a whole, in terms of money and disablement. In the USA alone it has been estimated that the annual cost of disease due to lost productivity, including medical care and disabled payments, may range from $222 to $1000 million. In the UK it has been estimated that four million working days are lost each year due to employees taking time off work because of skin disorders.

DEFINITION OF OCCUPATIONAL CONTACT DERMATITIS

Some countries have adopted a very strict definition of occupational contact dermatitis, whereas a broader definition is more useful. The American Medical Association's definition of 1939, 'An occupational dermatitis is a skin disease of which occupational exposure is a major causal or contributory factor,' encompasses the concept that work may also aggravate pre-existing skin conditions (1). Another more strict way of looking at whether or not a skin condition is occupational is to decide if the condition would have occurred even if the patient had not been doing the particular job in question.

Occupational contact dermatitis can occur at any age in a working life. There is widely thought to be a bimodal distribution of peaks in the incidence of dermatitis, the first occurring in the early years of the job and the second in middle age. In the younger age group it includes many patients with irritant and atopic dermatitis of the hands and in the older age group it is thought that the skin becomes progressively worn out by either an ageing process in the skin or through prolonged contact over many years, or a combination of the two (2).

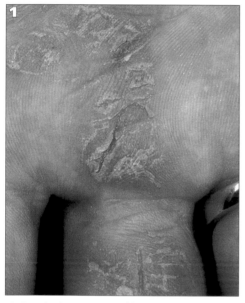

1 Psoriasis aggravated by manual work.

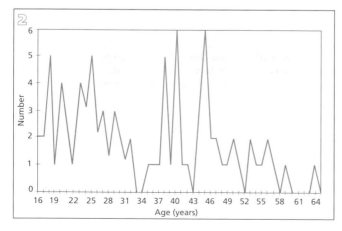

2 Onset of dermatitis in the pottery industry with age. There were peaks in the early twenties and mid-forties.

4

PROGNOSIS

Several studies have confirmed that the long-term prognosis for occupational contact dermatitis is often very bad. A Swedish study demonstrated that only 25% of 555 patients who had been investigated as having occupational contact dermatitis had completely healed over a 10 year period; one half still had periodic symptoms and one quarter permanent symptoms (3). Unfortunately, even for the 40% who changed their occupation, the overall prognosis was not improved (*Table 5*). Similarly, in a large follow-up study conducted in Western Australia, 55% of 949 patients still had dermatitis 2 years after the initial diagnosis.

It is not clear why the prognosis for occupational dermatitis is so poor though there are several explanations. The original cause may still be apparent or there may be contact with other causes either at home or in a different job, or, unfortunately, the chronicity of the dermatitis leads to inherent chronicity. It may be a combination of all three.

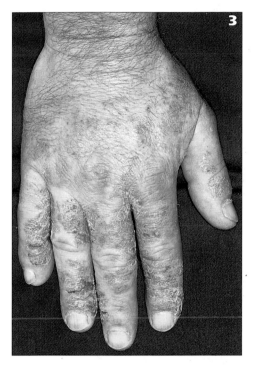

3 A chrome cripple. Sensitisation to potassium dichromate frequently leads to chronic dermatitis over many years. These patients are virtually unemployable and are severely disabled by dermatitis.

Table 5. The prognosis of occupational dermatitis is still bad even if there is a change in occupation; minimum follow-up 2 years.

Study	Number of patients	No change in job (% symptomatic)	Change in job (% symptomatic)
Western Australia (dermatitis from different occupations)	944	68	37
Soluble oil dermatitis	100	78	70
Catering dermatitis	32	79	69

AETIOLOGY

Contact dermatitis is often multifactorial. A constitutional tendency to atopy is a frequent finding (**4, 5**). Exposure to multiple irritants and allergens in a workplace is common, for example in hairdressing.

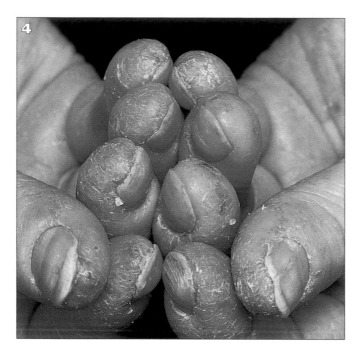

4 A chef had a type 1 allergy to monkfish, heavily infected finger eczema and an atopic background. His dermatitis was multifactorial in origin: allergic, irritant, constitutional factors and infection.

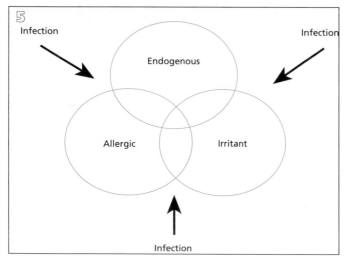

5 Frequently the causes of dermatitis are multifactorial.

PATTERNS OF CONTACT DERMATITIS

Most dermatologists accept that the final diagnosis cannot be predicted from the pattern of the dermatitis. Certain patterns of hand dermatitis used to be thought of as endogenous or more likely irritant or allergic, depending on the site. However, this is no longer accepted. There are few correlations in clinical patterns with aetiology (**6**) (see Chapter 6).

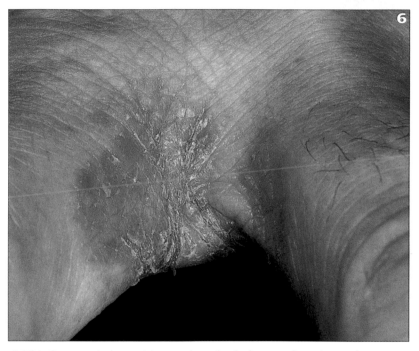

6 This finger web dermatitis was thought, before patch testing, to be irritant. The patient's patch tests showed a positive to Quaternium 15. The dermatitis cleared when the hand cleanser containing Quaternium 15 was removed from the patient's place of work, an engineering factory.

INVESTIGATIONS

Patients suffering from contact dermatitis should be thoroughly investigated to identify the allergens and/or irritants that may be causing their dermatitis. Irritants cannot be tested on the skin, except in order to exclude allergic causes – patch tests cannot determine whether or not the substance is irritant. Allergic contact dermatitis can be confirmed with patch tests; type 1 contact urticaria can be confirmed with scratch testing. Patch testing takes time and is difficult to do accurately (7), but its benefits are widely acknowledged to be essential for investigating a patient with dermatitis. The most important part of patch testing is interpreting the results, especially deciding whether they are false positive or false negative and their relevance. There are several commercially available patch series, in addition to the standard, that are useful in occupational contact dermatitis (*Table 6*).

Table 6. Additional patch series useful in the investigation of occupational dermatitis.

Series
Dental
Hairdressing
Isocyanates
Metal compounds
Meth(acrylate)
Oil and cooling fluid
Photographic chemicals
Glues and plastics
Textile colours and finishes

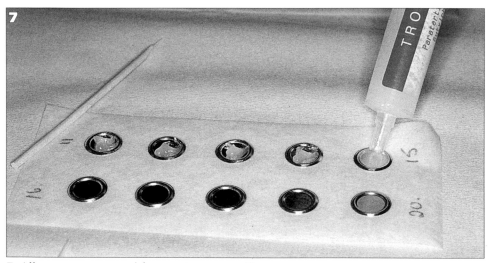

7 Allergens are squeezed from syringes on to Finn chambers prior to applying the patch tests.

PREVENTION

Pre-employment examination

Probably the most important aspect in a history for pre-employment screening is that of severe childhood eczema, especially with hand involvement. These people should be advised to avoid occupations such as those listed in *Table 7*.

Personal hygiene

To prevent is much better than to cure. Unfortunately, it is often very difficult to persuade workers, who have performed a job for years without any problems, that there is a risk of developing der-matitis until the dermatitis has actually occurred. Protective clothing, skin care products and skin cleansers should all be advised. It is well accepted that barrier creams are not very effective, however they do encourage the worker towards 'skin awareness'. Skin cleansers can also cause problems, either from allergy or irritancy (6).

Gloves are obviously essential in protecting the hands but it is also important to use gloves appropriate to the chemical with which the operative is in contact (*Table 8*). The regular use of an after-work emollient is probably the best way of reducing the chance of dermatitis occurring if contact with irritants cannot be avoided.

Table 7. At-risk occupations for irritant contact dermatitis.

Bakers
Butchers
Caterers
Cleaners
Construction workers
Food processors
Hairdressers
Horticulturists
Housewives/husbands
Masseurs
Metal workers
Motor mechanics
Nurses
Painters
Printers

Table 8. General guidance as to the suitability of various types of glove.

Material	Used against
Natural rubber	Soaps; detergents; water-soluble irritants; dilute acids and alkalis
Butyl rubber	Aldehydes; most amines; amides; ketones; formaldehyde resins; epoxy resins; most acrylates; isocyanates
Chloroprene	Soaps; detergents; dilute acids and alkalis; certain amines and esters; most alcohols; vegetable oils
Fluorocarbon	Organic solvents, particularly halogenated and aromatic hydrocarbons
Nitrile rubber	Organic acids; certain alcohols; amines; ethers; peroxides; inorganic alkalis; vegetable oils
Styrene–butadiene rubber	Bodily fluids hypoallergenic surgical gloves
Polyethylene	Used by food handlers and medical personnel
Polyvinyl alcohol	Several organic solvents; esters
Polyvinyl chloride	Soaps; detergents; oils; metalworking fluids; dilute acids and alkalis; vegetable oils

Workplace visit

Often when investigating a patient with contact dermatitis it is impossible to get the whole picture without visiting the patient's workplace. There are several indications for doing this:

- Detection of unexplained positive patch test.
- Detection of missed allergen.
- Substantiation of irritant contact dermatitis.
- Diagnosis of dermatoses in a workforce.
- Substantiation of non-occupational dermatoses.
- Industrial relations to calm the workforce's possible dermatological hysteria.

BIBLIOGRAPHY

Rycroft, RJG (1995), Occupational contact dermatitis, *Textbook of Contact Dermatitis*, Springer-Verlag, Berlin, 339–99.

CHAPTER TWO

IRRITANT CONTACT DERMATITIS

Chee Leok Goh

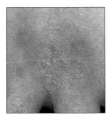

Irritant contact dermatitis is the most common presentation of occupational skin disease.

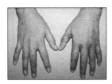

Soaps and detergents are common causes of irritant contact dermatitis.

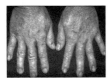

Dorsal pattern of dermatitis from cutting fluid.

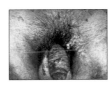

Acute irritant contact dermatitis from mustard gas.

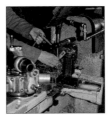

Automation of machines reduces the prevalence of contact dermatitis.

Chrome ulceration.

DEFINITION

Irritant contact dermatitis is defined as an inflammation of the skin resulting from a non-immunological reaction to external stimuli. These external stimuli are often skin irritants. Many industrial chemicals are potential skin irritants.

EPIDEMIOLOGY

Irritant contact dermatitis is the most common presentation of occupational skin disease. In industries where workers engage in wet work (e.g. food processing, hairdressing, cleaning, fishing industries), almost all workers develop some degree of irritant contact dermatitis. In the metal engineering industry more than 50% of workers who develop occupational skin diseases have irritant contact dermatitis. Most workers with mild occupational irritant contact dermatitis do not seek medical attention because the effect is usually not serious. They accept the condition as an occupational risk.

CLINICAL FEATURES

Classification of irritant skin reactions

Skin irritation from work chemicals can be classified into:
- Acute irritant reactions/burns.
- Irritant contact dermatitis:
  - acute irritant contact dermatitis.
  - chronic irritant contact dermatitis (cumulative insult dermatitis).
- Non-eczematous irritant reaction.

Acute irritant reactions/burns

Acute irritant reactions manifest as skin burns. The lesions are painful, red and oedematous. Erosions and skin ulcerations may occur (8, 9). The reaction is the result of direct chemical injury to the skin.

Common work chemicals that cause acute irritant reactions are given in the following list:
- Concentrated acids, e.g. sulphuric, nitric, hydrochloric, chromic and hydrofluoric.
- Strong alkalis, e.g. calcium, sodium and potassium hydroxides; wet concrete; sodium and potassium cyanides.
- Organic and inorganic salts, e.g. dichromates; arsenic salts.
- Solvents and gases, e.g. acrylonitrile; ethylene oxide; carbon disulphide; mustine.

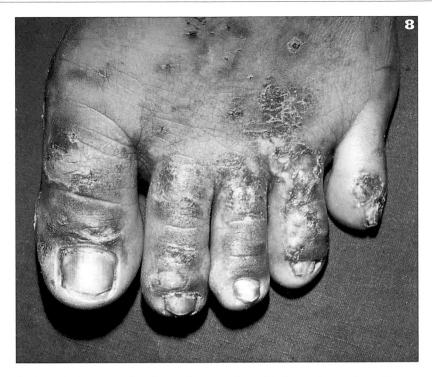

8 Acute irritant reaction: burns from gold cyanide in an electroplater. Note skin necrosis and erosions from the highly alkaline and toxic chemicals. Such an irritant reaction usually appears within hours of contact with the substance.

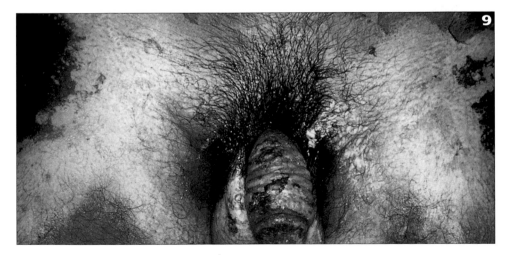

9 Nitrogen mustard gas burns in a soldier 2 weeks after exposure. Note the hyperpigmentation of some areas and that the groin has been affected.

Irritant contact dermatitis

The presentation of irritant contact dermatitis varies depending on the nature of the contact irritant and chronicity of exposure to the irritant. It may present as acute (**10, 11**) or chronic dermatitis (**12, 13**). This condition most commonly occurs on the dorsa of the hand and finger webs (**14, 15**).

Weak irritants, e.g. diluted acids, diluted alkalis, and solvents, are the commonest cause of irritant contact dermatitis. There is individual susceptibility to dif-

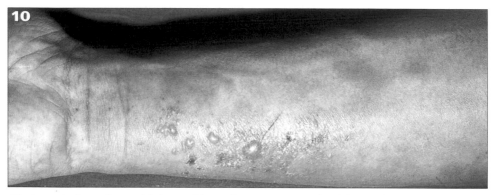

10 Acute irritant dermatitis in a solderer, from contact with soldering flux containing acids and alcohol. Note the vesiculation, erythema and oedema. Such reactions usually occur with strong irritants, e.g. acids and solvents.

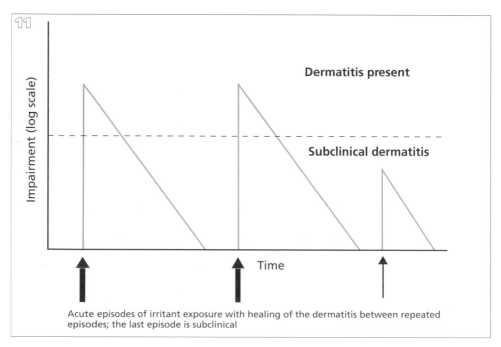

11 Graph showing episodes of acute irritant dermatitis.

ferent irritants as well as regional variability in terms of susceptibility. Clinically, irritant contact dermatitis is indistinguishable from allergic contact dermatitis. To differentiate between the two, a good occupational history, thorough physical examination and patch testing are necessary, though patch tests are only used for testing allergens and so negative results would be expected in irritant contact dermatitis. As yet there is no reliable human patch test to confirm irritant contact dermatitis; it is a diagnosis of exclusion with negative patch tests, knowing whether or not the substance is irritant and the degree of exposure to that irritant.

12 Chronic irritant contact dermatitis from prolonged exposure to water in an office cleaner. Note the dry, scaly, lichenified and fissured skin. This is a cumulative insult dermatitis resulting from extensive contact with water and detergents.

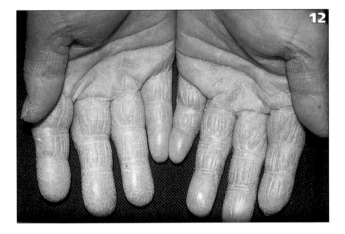

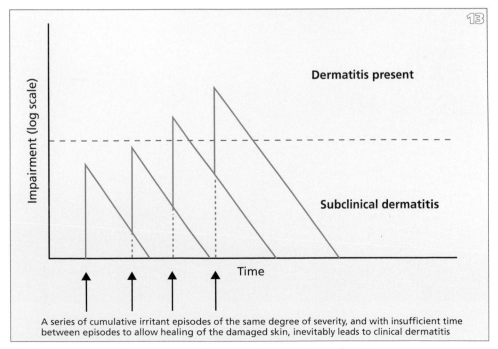

A series of cumulative irritant episodes of the same degree of severity, and with insufficient time between episodes to allow healing of the damaged skin, inevitably leads to clinical dermatitis

13 Graph showing the cumulative effect of subliminal doses of an irritant.

15

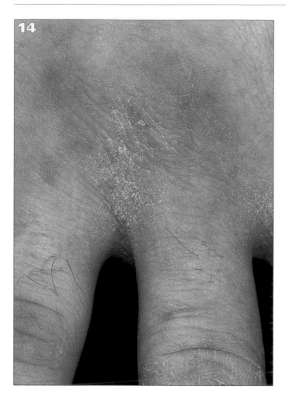

14, 15 The dorsa of the hands and the finger webs are the most common sites to be affected by irritant contact dermatitis but other areas such as fingers and palms can also be affected.

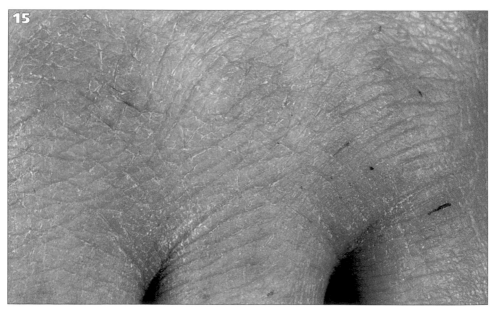

Acute irritant contact dermatitis

Itchy, vesiculo-erythematous and oede-matous eruptions occur after brief (few days) contact with irritant chemicals (10). Common causes of this type of dermatitis include moderate-to-weak acids, alkalis, soaps and detergents, solvents, metallic salts, cement, resins and cutting fluids.

Chronic irritant contact dermatitis (cumulative insult dermatitis)

Cumulative insult dermatitis presents as dry, scaly and fissuring eczematous patches on the fingers and hands. Fissuring and pigmentary changes may be present, but vesiculation is usually absent (12, 14, 15).

Common causes of cumulative insult dermatitis include weak irritants, e.g. water, skin cleanser (soaps and detergents), weak solvents and cutting fluids (13, 16).

At-risk occupations for cumulative insult dermatitis include those that involve wet work, e.g. chefs, bakers, bartenders, caterers, cleaners, hairdressers, metal workers, surgical nurses, printers, solderers, fisherman and construction workers.

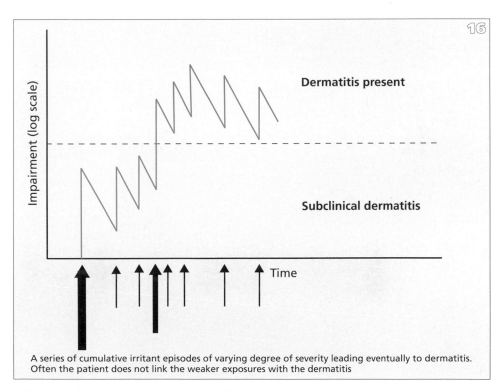

A series of cumulative irritant episodes of varying degree of severity leading eventually to dermatitis. Often the patient does not link the weaker exposures with the dermatitis

16 Graph showing a mixed causation of irritant contact dermatitis.

Non-eczematous irritant reactions

Some industrial chemicals and environments result in non-eczematous irritant reactions. These include folliculitis (17), miliaria (18), pigmentation, contact urticaria and granulomatous eruptions.

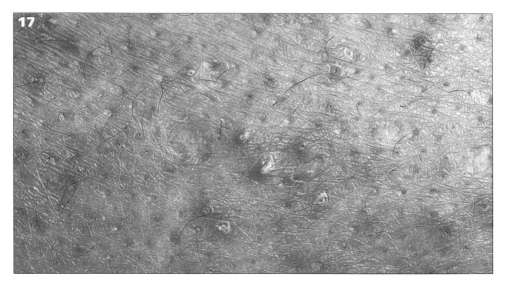

17 Oil folliculitis from contact with grease in a mechanic. Note the occlusion of the hair follicles with grease.

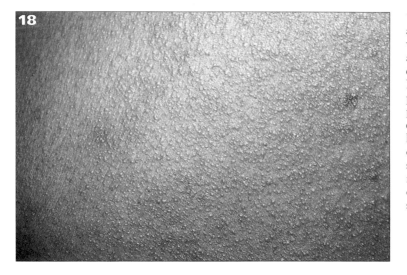

18 Miliaria on a boilerman working in a hot and humid environment. Note the pinhead-sized papular eruption. High humidity causes oedema of the sweat ducts resulting in obstruction and sweat retention.

MECHANISM OF IRRITANT CONTACT DERMATITIS

The pathogenic mechanism of acute irritant contact dermatitis is different to that of cumulative insult dermatitis.

In acute irritant contact dermatitis, the inflammatory reaction is mediated through the release of inflammatory mediators and cytokines. The reaction begins with the penetration of the irritant through the skin barrier and disruption of the cell membranes and lysosomes, resulting in inflammation. Some chemicals cause hyperaemia while others exhibit chemotactic activities. In acute irritant contact dermatitis, histologically there is spongiosis and mononuclear cell infiltration (lymphocytes and some monocytes) in the upper dermis (**19**). The histology of irritant contact dermatitis is generally indistinguishable from allergic contact dermatitis.

In cumulative insult dermatitis there is a slow disruption of the skin barrier (keratin layer and stratum corneum) which in turn stimulates an increase in epidermal turnover leading to dryness, scaliness and lichenification. Damage to the lipid barrier of the skin is associated with loss of cohesion of corneocytes causing desquamation.

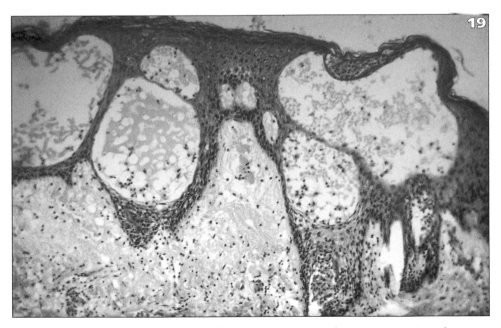

19 Histology of acute irritant contact dermatitis. Note vesiculation, spongiosis and mononuclear cell infiltration in the dermis.

The intercellular lipids of the stratum corneum appear to play an important part in the barrier function of the skin. Ceramides and glycosylceramides appear to be the key elements in maintaining the water retention properties of the stratum corneum. The whole process triggers lipid synthesis, proliferation of keratinocytes, transient hyperkeratosis and restoration of the skin barrier. Histologically, lesions of cumulative insult dermatitis show hyperkeratosis and acanthosis in addition to the mononuclear infiltration in the upper dermis (20).

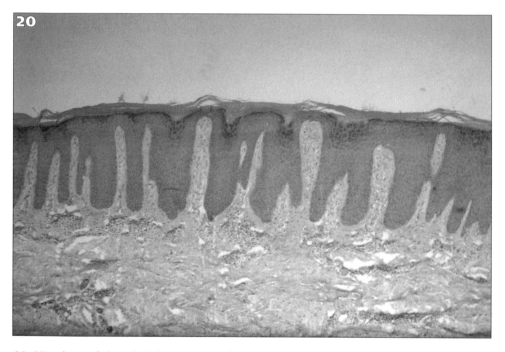

20 Histology of chronic irritant contact dermatitis. Note the hyperkeratosis, acanthosis and mononuclear infiltrate in the upper dermis.

PREDISPOSING AND RISK FACTORS

Different subjects develop different degrees of irritation when exposed to the same irritants under the same conditions. Different parts of the body also have different susceptibilities to the same irritants under similar conditions. Factors that influence individual susceptibility include age, site, race, gender and past history of dermatitis.

Age and site

Skin susceptibility to the irritant effects of surfactants appears to decrease with age. Studies have shown that skin irritability to sodium lauryl sulphate (using trans-epidermal water loss measurements) peaks during childhood and declines steadily during adult life, reaching its lowest value by the sixth decade of life. Sites with the greatest reactivity due to age were the thigh, upper back and forearm.

Race

Darker-skinned individuals, such as of African origin and Hispanics, show a higher irritation response to the surfactant sodium lauryl sulphate, which suggests a different reaction of darker skin to irritants.

Gender

There is no difference in susceptibility to skin irritation between the genders. However, studies have indicated that female skin tends to be more susceptible to irritation during the pre-menstrual period.

Pre-existing dermatitis and atopic dermatitis

Subjects with a history of dermatitis appear to be more susceptible to the irritant effects of sodium lauryl sulphate compared to controls. Trans-epidermal water loss (TEWL) is higher in subjects with a positive history of dermatitis after exposure to different concentrations of sodium lauryl sulphate. Studies have also shown that normal, uninvolved and atopic skin behaves differently from non-atopic skin in having a higher baseline TEWL and decreased stratum corneum water content. A reduction in ceramides associated with structural alterations of the stratum corneum has also been demonstrated in the skin of patients with atopic dermatitis. Abnormalities of the barrier in the skin of atopic individuals may be an important factor behind the increased susceptibility of atopic skin to irritation.

Xerosis

Skin with marked xerosis tends to induce higher TEWL responses after application of sodium lauryl sulphate at different concentrations indicating an increased susceptibility of xerotic skin to irritants.

Diagnostic test

There is no simple and reliable diagnostic test for individual susceptibility to skin irritation. The diagnosis of irritant contact dermatitis is based on a detailed history, clinical examination and exclusion of allergic contact dermatitis by patch testing.

21

COMMON OCCUPATIONAL IRRITANTS

Water, detergents and soaps

Soaps and detergents are commonly used skin cleansers, used by all workers in all industries; they are generally weak skin irritants. Excessive skin cleansing with soaps and detergents causes cumulative insult dermatitis in predisposed individuals. At-risk groups are workers in the cleaning, food/catering and construction industries, hairdressers, and hospital workers.

Soaps and detergents are skin irritants because they contain weak alkalis, emulsifiers, surfactants and sometimes enzymes. Irritant contact dermatitis from soaps and detergents usually begins in the finger webs and on the skin under rings (**21**). The dermatitis tends to spread to the adjacent finger shaft, the dorsum of the hand and the palms. Paronychia and nail dystrophy are not uncommon. Workers with a history of atopic eczema or hand eczema are particularly predisposed to the irritant effects of soaps and detergents.

Acids and alkalis

Acids and alkalis are used in various industrial processes as solvents and cleansers. Commonly used industrial acids include hydrochloric, nitric, sulphuric, chromic, hydrofluoric and acetic. Commonly used industrial alkalis include sodium, potassium and calcium hydroxides, ammonia, sodium carbonate and amines. Acids and alkalis are commonly used in electroplating processes and by floor-layers, masons, jewellers and tanners. Chromic acid, used in the chrome-plating process, is a strong skin irritant and causes burns (**22**) and irritant contact dermatitis.

Inorganic cyanide, e.g. gold cyanide used in electroplating, is a strong alkali causing severe burns (**8**).

Hydrofluoric acid is used by construction workers. It is a strong acid causing severe tissue necrosis. Progressive necrosis continues for several days, even after the wound has been thoroughly cleansed (**23**).

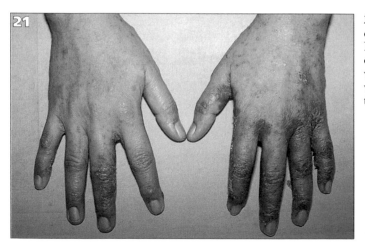

21 Irritant contact dermatitis from soaps. Note the eczema occurring under the wedding ring, finger webs and spreading to the adjacent fingers.

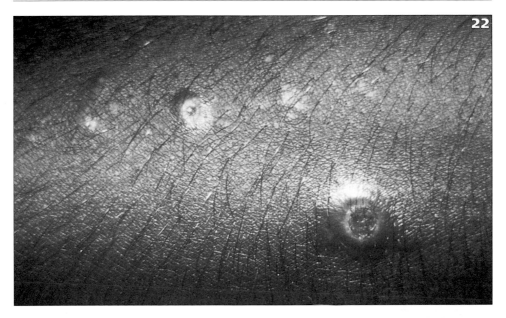

22 Chrome ulcer: acute skin erosions from chromic acid burns. Note the round, discrete punched out lesions. Perforation of the nasal septum and palate may also occur.

23 Hydrofluoric acid burns. Note the severe tissue necrosis and erythema. Such necrosis tends to progress even after the wound has been cleansed.

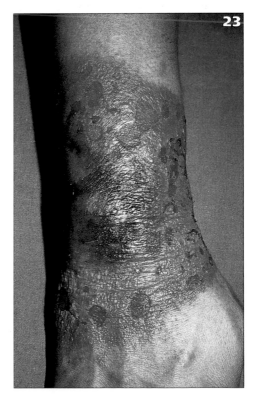

Cement

Wet cement is strongly alkaline (because of its limestone content) and is an irritant, causing cement burns and irritant contact dermatitis. Cement burns present as erosive skin lesions on pressure areas of the limbs (24). Repeated contact with wet cement can lead to cumulative insult dermatitis.

Solvents

Solvents are liquids capable of dissolving various substances. They are used as dilutants in adhesives, paints, inks and pharmaceutical products, as carriers of other chemicals and for degreasing in many manufacturing processes.

Common industrial solvents include aliphatic and aromatic hydrocarbons such as alcohol, formalin, kerosene, toluene, xylene, benzene, ethers, ketones, amines and chlorinated hydrocarbons.

Solvents are degreasing agents and tend to cause acute irritant contact dermatitis and cumulative insult dermatitis. They cause physical damage to the protective keratin and stratum corneum layer of the skin leading to epidermal dehydration; volatile solvents may cause airborne dermatitis. Solvent irritant dermatitis usually occurs on the fingers where contact is most intense.

Soldering fluxes

Soldering fluxes are solvents containing alcohol, glacial acetic acid, amines and other chemicals. They are used to clean metallic surfaces during soldering especially in the electronics and electrical industries; soldering flux is the commonest cause of irritant contact dermatitis in the electronics industry. Dermatitis usually occurs on the finger

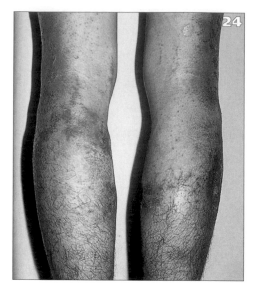

24 Cement burns. Note the erosive lesions from the alkaline burn. Cement burns tend to occur on pressure areas, e.g. the knees, ankles and skin folds.

pulps spreading to the finger shafts (25). It is a cause of acute irritant and cumulative insult dermatitis. Cotton gloves worn by solderers often have a wick effect in absorbing the flux during work, enhancing the effect of the irritant on the skin of the fingers.

Fibreglass

Fibreglass is widely used as an insulator in electrical appliances and air-conditioner ducts. It is also commonly used in furniture and ceiling board. It is an important component of printed circuit boards.

Fibreglass consists of sharp glass spicules (26) capable of penetrating the superficial part of the horny layer of the skin, which causes immediate skin irritation. The acute irritation reaction results in pruriginous eruptions (27). Clothing may trap the fibreglass and cause pruriginous dermatitis on covered parts of the body.

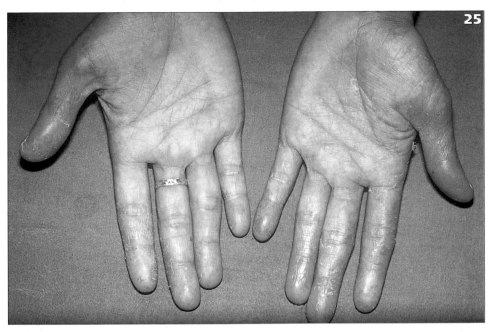

25 Chronic irritant contact dermatitis in a solderer from soldering flux. The flux contains alcohol, glacial acetic acid, amines and other chemicals. It is a skin irritant. Note the dry, scaly dermatitis affecting most fingers due to contamination from wet cotton gloves.

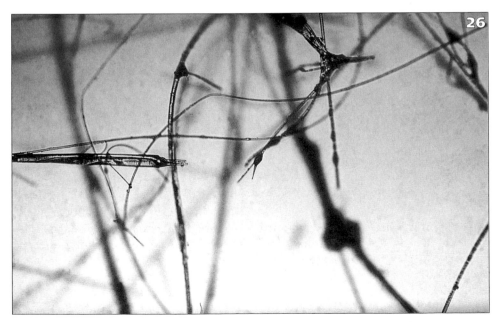

26 Fibreglass under magnification. Note the sharp spicules which are capable of penetrating the superficial horny layer of the skin to cause irritation.

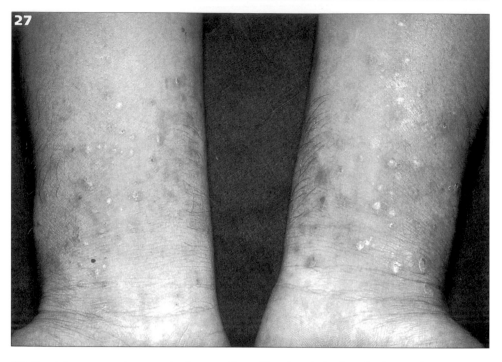

27 Pruriginous eruptions on the forearm from fibreglass irritation. Such eruptions may occur on covered areas of the body due to airborne contamination.

Cutting fluids

Cutting fluids are used daily in the metal and optical industries for lubrication and cooling during cutting, grinding and lathe operations. Various types of cutting are used fluids, which include soluble and insoluble oils. Synthetic, water-soluble oils appear to cause more skin irritation than do neat mineral oils (28).

Irritant contact dermatitis is common among metalworkers in contact with cutting fluids. It usually occurs after prolonged and repeated contact with the fluids, often on the dorsum of the fingers and hands. The morphology is commonly that of discoid eczema over bony prominences, e.g. the knuckles and interphalangeal joints (29).

Foods

Uncooked food causes irritant contact dermatitis in food handlers and chefs. Cumulative insult dermatitis results from prolonged contact with water, and the enzymes and alkaloids present in some foodstuffs including meat and vegetables. Irritant contact dermatitis in chefs is often associated with paronychia (see Chapter 12).

28 Soluble oil is used to cool the components being machined. Direct prolonged contact of the skin of operatives still occurs in some factories but greater automation is reducing the incidence of irritant contact dermatitis.

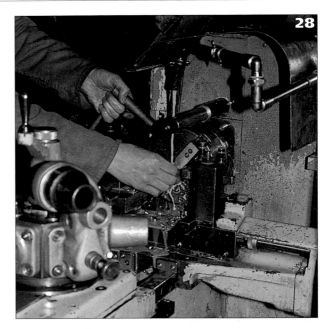

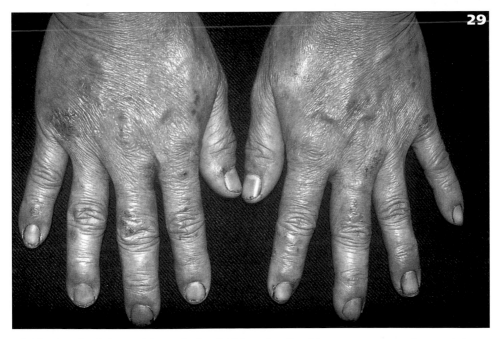

29 Cutting fluid dermatitis on the hands. Note the discoid eczematous eruptions mainly over the bony prominences of the hands. This is usually the result of cumulative insult dermatitis. Most workers working with cutting fluids develop this dermatitis.

TREATMENT AND PREVENTION

Treatment

In acute weeping dermatitis, wet compresses with normal saline or diluted potassium permanganate or Burrow's solution help to clear wet, oozing eczematous lesions. Topical corticosteroids remain the cornerstone in the treatment of irritant contact dermatitis; systemic steroids may be indicated in acute dermatitis. Secondary infection should be treated with a systemic antibiotic and a topical steroid combined with an antibiotic–antiseptic preparation.

Prevention

All irritant contact dermatitis is preventable. Most workers are able to return to their work after treatment and rehabilitation. Workers should be educated on various preventative measures against this dermatitis before starting work, such as good occupational hygiene and working practice. Another preventative measure is to use effective pre-employment screening.

Pre-employment screening

Workers with underling predisposing factors (such as atopic dermatitis, hand eczema or xerosis) should avoid wet work and employment exposing them to irritants, e.g. solvents, acids and alkali. These workers should be identified and counselled to change to dry work. Pre-employment identification of at-risk individuals and early job counselling may prevent the occurrence of irritant contact dermatitis in susceptible people.

Workplace

Clean workplace

Contamination of the workbench and inadequate cleansing facilities are common causes of irritant contact dermatitis. Workers should be encouraged to maintain a clean and well-ventilated working environment.

Washing facilities and skin cleansers

Management should ensure adequate washing facilities and appropriate skin cleansers. Workers should not use abrasive skin cleansers and be discouraged from degreasing the skin with organic solvents and abrasive detergents.

Gloves, boots and aprons

Workers should be required to wear proper protective gloves, boots and aprons where indicated. These should be provided by the management.

Barrier creams

By themselves, barrier creams are of questionable value against irritant contact dermatitis. Their use should not be over promoted as this will give workers a false sense of security and encourage them to be complacent in implementing the appropriate preventative measures.

After-work emollients

These creams appear to confer some degree of protection against irritant contact dermatitis. They should be encouraged and made available in the workplace.

Health education

Health education is probably the most important aspect in the prevention of occupational skin disease. New workers should be educated on the causes and preventative measures against occupational dermatitis. Workers should be informed on the hazards of the work process and work chemicals. Health education should be incorporated into the curriculum of workers' training programmes.

Irritant contact dermatitis is often the result of multiple factors including occupational and non-occupational contact factors and underlying endogenous factors (see Chapter 1).

In managing patients with occupational irritant contact dermatitis it is important to identify any non-occupational causes that may be potential aggravating factors. This includes the avoidance of irritants at home and in hobbies.

BIBLIOGRAPHY

Frosch, PJ (1995), Cutaneous irritation, *Textbook of Contact Dermatitis*, Springer-Verlag, Berlin, 28–61.

Malten, KE (1981), Thoughts on irritant contact dermatitis, *Contact Dermatitis*; 7: 435–8.

CHAPTER THREE

ALLERGIC CONTACT DERMATITIS: IMMUNOLOGICAL ASPECTS AND COMMON OCCUPATIONAL CAUSES

Neils K Veien

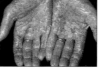

Immediate type 1 hypersensitivity reactions can be demonstrated with scratch testing.

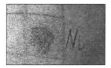

Delayed type 4 allergic hypersensitivity is confirmed by patch testing and reading at 48 and 96 hours.

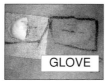

All patients with chronic hand eczema should be patch tested.

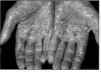

Eyelid eczema is caused commonly by allergic contact dermatitis.

DELAYED-TYPE HYPERSENSITIVITY

The skin has an important function at the periphery of the human immune system – a first line of defence. The reaction pattern known as allergic contact dermatitis is a prototype of a delayed-type hypersensitivity reaction. Such reactions effectively combat invasive micro-organisms. Allergic contact dermatitis can be thought of as the exaggerated reaction pattern of an effective defence system.

Sensitisation

Haptens of low molecular weight that penetrate the skin bind to antigen-presenting, epidermal Langerhan's cells at the site of contact. This binding is secured by a number of cellular adhesion molecules. The Langerhan's cells travel to the regional lymph nodes where naïve T-cells become sensitised to the hapten in question. These sensitised T-cells enter the circulatory system and are distributed throughout the body, thus sensitising the entire surface of the skin (30).

The sensitisation capacity of different haptens varies greatly with a number of individual factors contributing to the fact that one person may become sensitised to a substance, while another, faced with the same exposure, does not. There is also an individual variability in a person's capacity to become sensitised.

Sensitisation to common haptens which regularly stimulate the immune system is lifelong, while sensitisation to haptens with which contact is rare may fade over time. There is some evidence that tolerance can be induced by repeated oral exposure to a hapten in already sensitised persons and also that this method can be used to prevent sensitisation.

Elicitation

In sensitised persons, skin contact with a hapten results in penetration, antigen binding and presentation via the Langerhan's cells, as described above. When an antigen is presented to specifically sensitised T-lymphocytes in the dermis, these will release a number of cytokines, the cytokines then attracting other sensitised T-lymphocytes and other

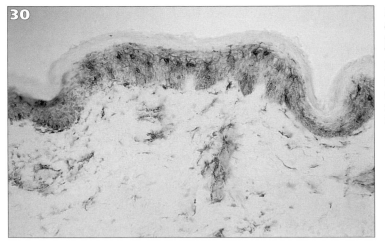

30 Langerhan's cells are found in the mid-epidermis. They identify haptens and present them to the cell-mediated mechanisms of the immune system.

31 A true-positive patch test to nickel.

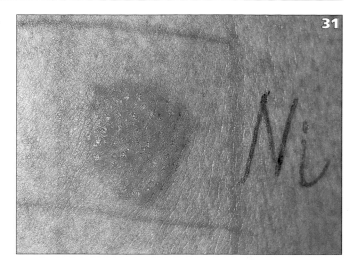

types of leukocytes. The ensuing vasodilation and cellular interaction results in the epidermal and dermal inflammation clinically described as an eczematous reaction (31). The length of time from contact with the hapten to the appearance of a clinically identifiable reaction is 1–3 days.

Patch testing is the principal diagnostic procedure used to identify the cause of allergic contact dermatitis. In principle, a patch test reaction is a reproduction of the elicitation phase of allergic contact dermatitis and is obtained by placing a small amount of the suspected hapten on the skin. The test is uncomplicated and cheap.

Over the past 50 years, standardised test substances in optimal concentrations and suitable vehicles have been developed. There are, however, a number of pitfalls in the patch testing procedure. Interpretation of the test results requires considerable skill, and care must be taken to minimise the risk of false-positive readings. There is also a risk of false-negative reactions. A true positive patch test typically showing erythema, papules or vesicles, is infiltrated and spreads beyond

the test site (31). An irritant reaction, on the other hand, is sharply demarcated and shows erythema, little infiltration and pustules (32). Non-specific hyper-reaction or 'angry back' is often seen if the test is performed when the dermatitis is very active or if a patient with atopic dermatitis is tested with metals.

Special series of patch test substances are available all over the world from several suppliers. The series should reflect geographical variations in products to

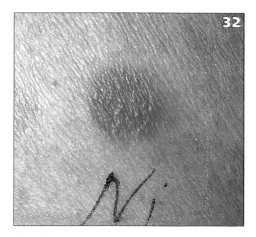

32 A false-positive patch test to nickel.

which the local population is ordinarily exposed. The European standard series of allergens is shown in *Table 9*.

The most important occupational allergens include chromate, cobalt, nickel, epoxy resin, formaldehyde and formaldehyde resins, acrylates, fragrances, plants and rubber additives.

IMMEDIATE-TYPE HYPERSENSITIVITY

High molecular weight antigens such as proteins may induce specific IgE antibody production. Many of these antigens can only penetrate thin skin or a defective skin surface. If the antigen and specific IgE antibodies bind to Fc receptors on the mast cells, these will release histamine and other mediators. The typical clinical picture is an urticarial reaction with erythema and oedema. Contact urticaria can be an occupational dermatosis if caused, for example, by latex in rubber gloves (33). Veterinarians exposed to amniotic fluid (34) and kitchen staff who have contact with uncooked food may develop protein contact dermatitis, a variant of contact urticaria (35, 36).

Allergic contact dermatitis can be the cause of occupational dermatoses in a variety of occupations. Those in which the incidence of allergic contact dermatitis is relatively high include cement casters, construction workers, printers and graphics workers, farmers, gardeners, painters, woodworkers, hospital employees, cleaners and workers in the electronics and food processing industries.

Table 9. The European standard series of allergens is the most widely used patch test series. Many dermatologists will adapt the series to suit the local population's exposure to various allergens.

Potassium dichromate
Neomycin sulphate
Thiuram mix
p-phenylenediamine
Cobalt chloride
Benzocaine
Formaldehyde
Colophony
Quinoline mix
Balsam of Peru
PPD–black rubber mix
Wool alcohols (lanolin)
Mercapto mix
Epoxy resin
Paraben mix
Butylphenol–formaldehyde resin
Fragrance mix
Quaternium 15
Nickel sulphate
Isothiazolinones
Mercaptobenzothiazole
Primin
Sesquiterpene lactone mix

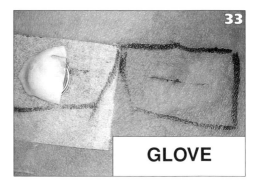

33 A positive scratch-chamber test with a latex glove. A superficial scratch in the skin covered with a piece of latex will cause an urticarial reaction in 15–20 minutes.

34 The forearms of
a veterinary surgeon
after delivery of a
calf.

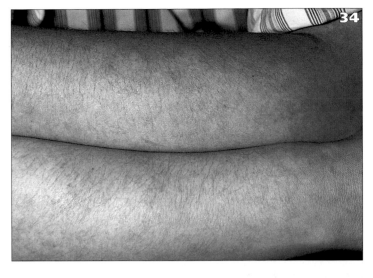

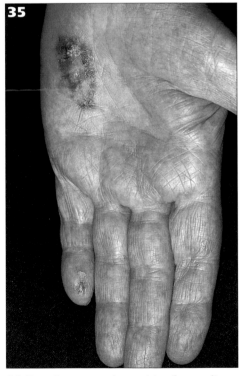

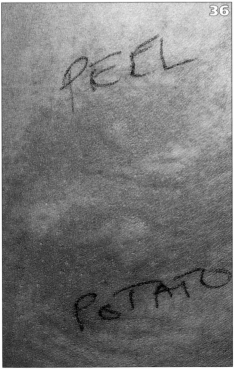

35 Protein contact dermatitis after peeling
a raw potato.

36 A positive prick test to potato peel (top
half) and potato pulp (bottom half).

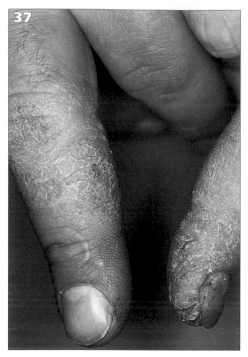

37 Allergic contact dermatitis of the fingers.

CLINICAL FEATURES

Hand dermatitis is the most frequently seen occupational allergic contact dermatitis. This is commonly seen on the dorsal aspects of the hands and in the finger webs, presumably because allergens can easily penetrate the thin skin at these sites (37, 38). The forearms of patients with hand dermatitis are often also involved (39). Fingertip dermatitis is characteristic of chefs allergic to garlic (40, 41, 42, 43) and among dental employees sensitive to acrylates. Nail dystrophy with multiple transversal depressions like Beau lines may be seen if hand eczema involves the periungual area (44).

Airborne allergens like those present in some types of plant dust may cause dermatitis of the face, neck and arms (45).

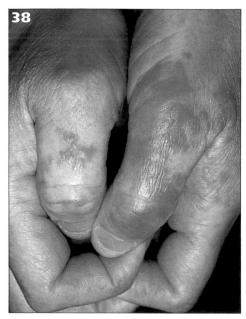

38 Allergic contact dermatitis of the hands and fingers.

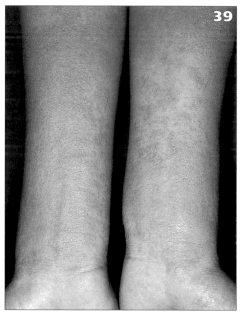

39 Allergic contact dermatitis from rubber gloves.

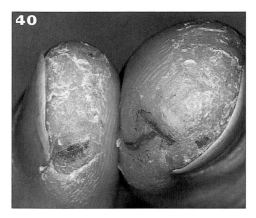

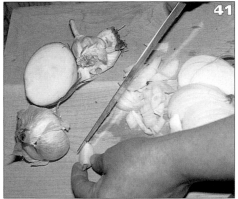

40 Fingertip dermatitis on the thumb and first finger on the left hand of a chef.

41 In a right-handed person the garlic is held in the left hand and the knife in the right, hence the dermatitis is usually confined to the thumb and the tip of the first finger of the left hand.

42 Patch test with 50% garlic in arachis oil. A sliver of garlic, or some of it crushed, can be irritant on patch testing.

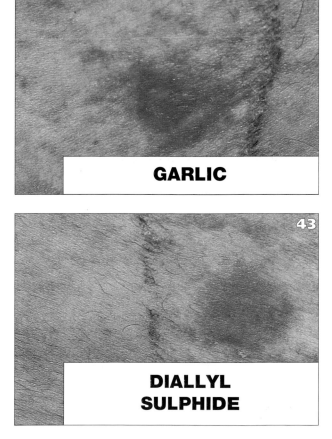

43 The allergen causing garlic contact dermatitis is diallyl sulphide.

37

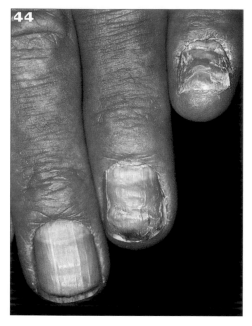

44 'Eczema nails' in a patient with chronic hand dermatitis.

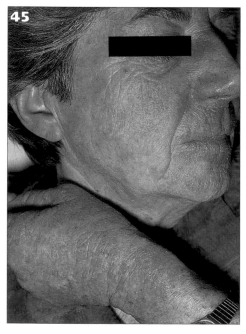

45 Airborne allergic contact dermatitis from Compositae plants.

COMMON CAUSES OF ALLERGIC CONTACT DERMATITIS

Typically affected occupations are noted in the following overview of allergens commonly responsible for allergic contact dermatitis.

Chromate

While metallic chromium does not sensitise, hexavalent chromates readily penetrate the skin and are common contact sensitisers, particularly amongst men. Allergic contact dermatitis caused by chromate can result in severe hand eczema in builders (46); the allergic reaction is caused by dichromates in cement. The addition of ferrous sulphate to cement reduces hexavalent chromium to trivalent chromium which is a poor skin penetrator and rarely elicits allergic contact dermatitis in chromate-sensitive persons. Dichromates are also used as leather tanning agents, and contact patterns of dermatitis may appear after contact with leather safety shoes and wooden shoes with leather tops worn at work (47). Other sources of occupational exposure to chromates include wood preservatives, magnetic tapes, anti-corrosive agents, welding fumes and fire retardants.

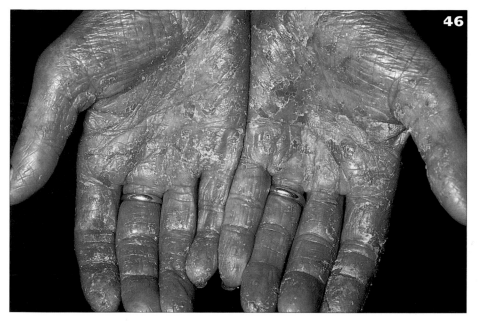

46 Chromate dermatitis.

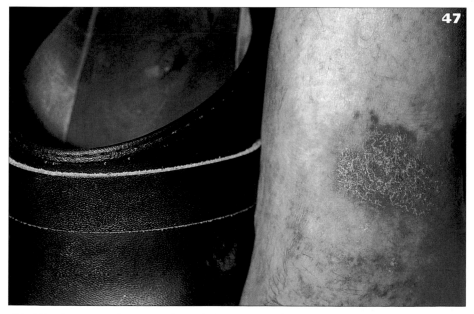

47 Allergic contact dermatitis from dichromate used in tanning leather.

Cobalt

The metal cobalt is used in various types of hardened steel. Nickel is often contaminated with cobalt, and cobalt allergy is common in women who are sensitive to nickel. In men, cobalt allergy is often associated with chromate allergy. Non-metallic sources of exposure to cobalt are the blue pigments used for painting pottery and china and siccantives in varnish and paint (48).

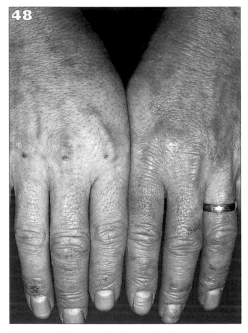

48 Hand dermatitis in a cobalt-sensitive patient who had spray-painted his bicycle with a blue paint containing cobalt.

Nickel

This is the most common contact sensitiser in most countries. Approximately 10% of women and 1% of men in industrialised countries are nickel sensitive. The sensitisation is predominantly non-occupational and is caused by skin contact with non-precious metals (49).

The presence of nickel in metal objects in amounts sufficient to elicit allergic nickel dermatitis is easily demonstrated by the nickel spot test. Solutions of ammonium hydroxide and sodium dimethylglyoxime are dropped onto a cotton-tipped applicator which is then rubbed against the object suspected to contain nickel. If the item releases nickel in an amount equal to more than 0.5 µg/cm², the spot that has been rubbed will turn bright red (50). Whether or not the hands of a patient are exposed to nickel in clean workplaces can be demonstrated if the patient wears cotton gloves during working hours. The dimethylglyoxime test can then be applied to the gloves (51).

Elicitation of the dermatitis in sensitised persons can be caused by occupational contact with nickel used, for example, in the nickel-plating and electronics industries (52) or by the use of safety footwear with buttons containing nickel (53). Frequent or regular contact with coins that contain nickel may cause dermatitis on the fingers (54). In spite of the 10% nickel content in many stainless steels, dermatitis in nickel-sensitive persons is not caused by this alloy because the nickel is tightly bound. In addition to nickel-plated items or alloys containing nickel, salts of the metal are used in some batteries, pigments and catalysts.

49 The most common cause of nickel allergic contact dermatitis is from metal jewellery or watch-straps.

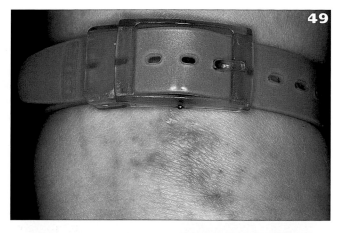

50 A watch-strap giving a positive dimethylglyoxime test for nickel.

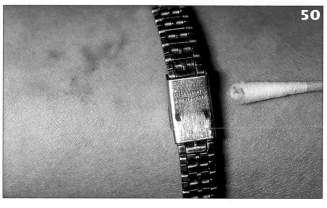

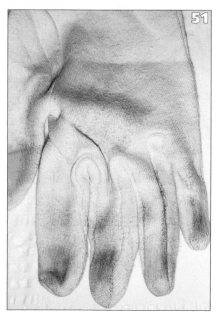

51 A positive dimethylglyoxime test on gloves after a day's work in the electronics industry.

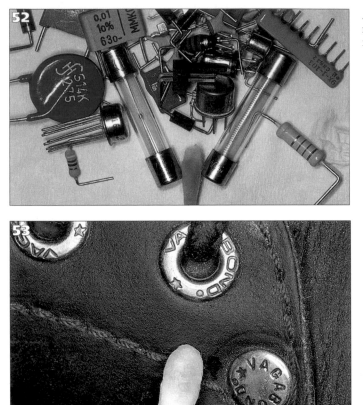

52 Electrical components are a rich source for nickel contact.

53 Even buckles on safety shoes are likely to contain nickel.

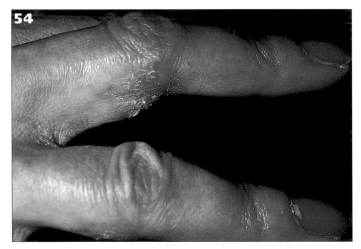

54 Handling coins frequently during the day worsened this woman's dermatitis.

Rubber

Rubber items may cause allergic contact dermatitis due to their content of vulcanisers and anti-oxidants. Rubber additives that are common sensitisers include thiurams and carbamates, used in a wide variety of moulded rubber items such as latex gloves (55). Rubber additives used especially in footwear include mercaptobenzothiazole and similar chemical compounds (56, 57). Weather-resistant black rubber compounds such as car tyres contain the anti-oxidant IPPD (4-isopropylaminodiphenylamine) and other derivatives of phenylenediamine.

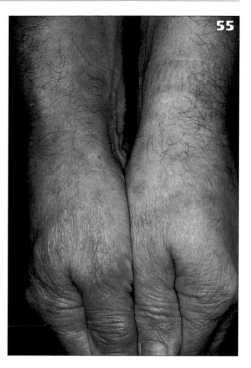

55 Allergic contact dermatitis from thiuram-containing rubber gloves. Thiuram is an additive used in the manufacturing process of rubber gloves.

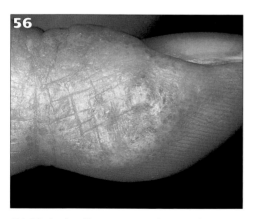

56 Vesicular finger eczema in a patient who wore heavy-duty rubber gloves containing mercaptobenzothiazole as a vulcaniser.

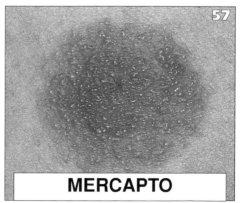

MERCAPTO

57 The patient described in 56 reacted positively to mercapto mix.

Latex may cause immunological contact urticaria due to the formation of specific IgE antibodies. The clinical picture may include an urticarial reaction on the dorsal aspects of the hands of sensitised persons who wear rubber gloves. A saline extract of the rubber glove can be made in a few minutes and used for prick testing (58).

Formaldehyde

This is present in many cosmetics, some plastics and in some types of paper. Biocides used in cutting oil and water soluble paint may release formaldehyde. A positive patch test to formaldehyde in men with hand eczema is usually occupational in origin.

Colophony

This is the sticky substance exuded by pine trees. It is used in manufacturing paper, glue and sticking plaster, in various sports to improve grip and in the printing industry. Fingertip dermatitis (59) was seen in a colophony-sensitive radiography technician who handled envelopes (60). Patch test application of the envelope paper produced a positive reaction (61). Dermatitis at sites where adhesives have been applied is often due to colophony sensitivity (62).

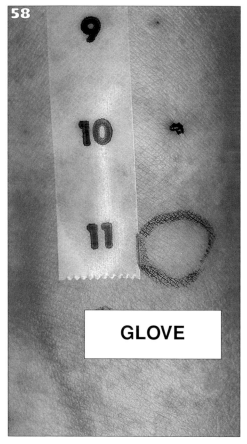

58 A positive prick test to latex solution.

59 Fingertip dermatitis from colophony in radiograph envelopes.

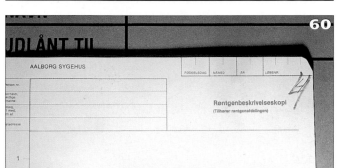

60 Paper is manufactured from fir tree pulp which contains colophony.

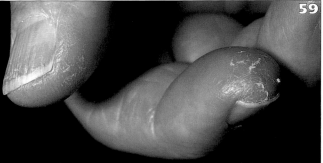

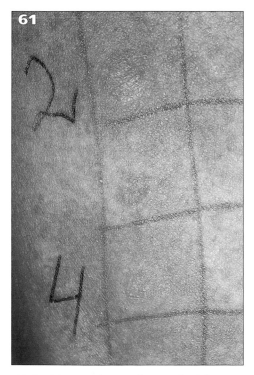

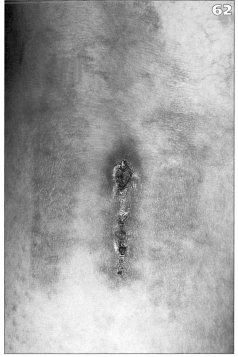

61 Positive patch tests that resulted from a radiograph envelope.

62 The most common cause of colophony sensitivity is from sticking plaster.

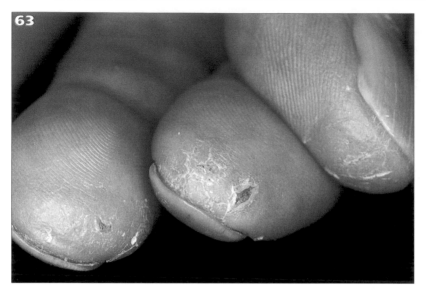

63 Fingertip dermatitis in a dental assistant caused by acrylates.

Acrylates

A wide variety of acrylates are used as adhesives and sealants in industry and in dentistry. Fingertip dermatitis caused by acrylates is seen in dentists and dental assistants (63).

Epoxy

Patients sensitive to epoxy may experience severe dermatitis at the site of contact (64) and very commonly will spread to involve the eyelids either by direct contact or by fumes (65). The epoxy resin

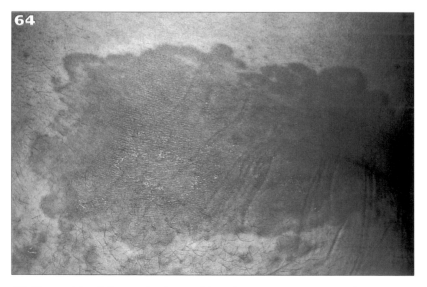

64 Dermatitis of the trunk after accidental exposure to epoxy resin.

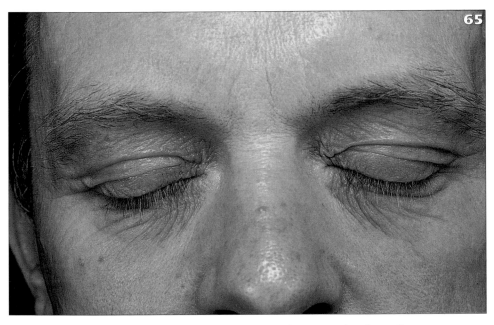

65 Epoxy resin dermatitis in a patient using epoxy adhesives to lay floor tiles.

is usually the sensitiser but hardeners and reactive diluents can also sensitise.

Fragrances

Fragrances are common sensitisers, largely due to the wide use of scented products in the home. Occupational allergic contact dermatitis caused by scented detergents and cleaning agents are commonly seen on the hands and face (66).

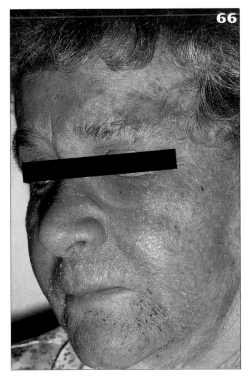

66 Facial dermatitis in a fragrance-sensitive cleaner.

Plants

Allergic contact dermatitis from plants is an occupational hazard among florists, gardeners and farmers (see Chapter 7). Striped patterns of dermatitis are characteristic (**67**). Oedematous hand dermatitis was seen in a florist who had arranged *Alstroemeria* (**68, 69**). *Primula obconica* contains the strongly sensitising primin (2-methoxy-6-pentylbenzoquinone) (**70, 71**). The *Compositae* family of plants (**72**) contains sesquiterpene lactones, compounds which are highly sensitising; an airborne pattern of dermatitis is typical. This dermatitis may evolve into the actinic reticuloid syndrome (**73**).

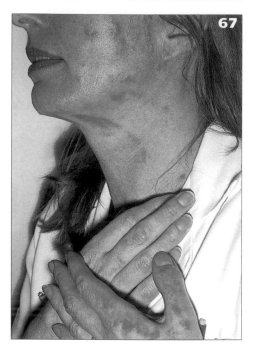

67 Allergic contact dermatitis from plants often causes striped patterns of dermatitis.

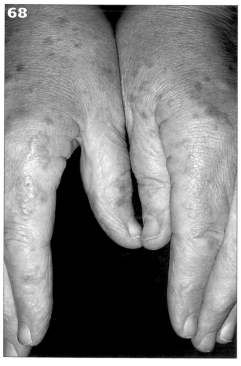

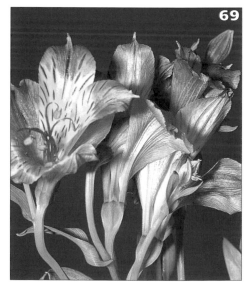

68 Oedematous hand dermatitis in a florist who had arranged *Alstroemeria*.

69 *Alstroemeria*.

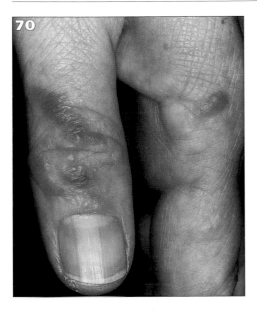

70 Primula dermatitis is often bullous and severe. The linear lesions are characteristic of plant dermatitis.

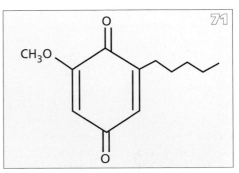

71 Chemical structure of primin.

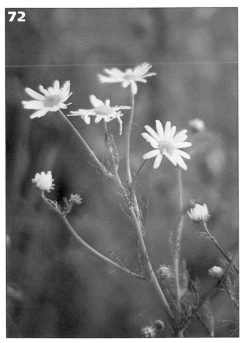

72 The *Compositae* family of plants contain sesquiterpene lactones.

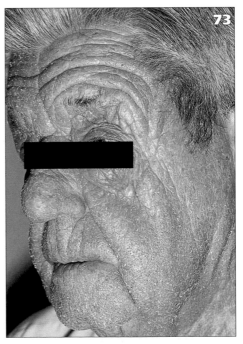

73 These compounds are highly sensitising; an airborne pattern of dermatitis is typical. This dermatitis may evolve into the actinic reticuloid syndrome.

Other sensitisers

Hairdressers may become sensitised to thioglycolates in perm solutions, to the hair dye *p*-phenylenediamine or to ammonium persulphate used to bleach

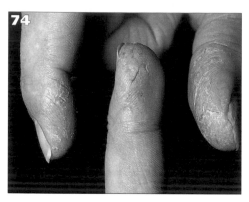

74 Handling vials containing antibiotics caused fingertip dermatitis.

hair. Immediate- as well as delayed-type hypersensitivity may be seen following contact with ammonium persulphate.

Farmers come into contact with a number of sensitisers when, for example, pigs are treated with antibiotics; the handling of vials containing antibiotics may cause fingertip dermatitis (74). Another clinical picture seen among farmers is airborne dermatitis caused by dust contaminated with antibiotics (75).

Allergic contact urticaria from food items such as tomatoes, potatoes and cheese is common among sandwich makers. The characteristic symptoms are stinging, pruritus and pain occurring seconds to minutes after contact with the offending substance. Repeated contact with flour and dough can cause protein contact dermatitis in bakers (76, 77).

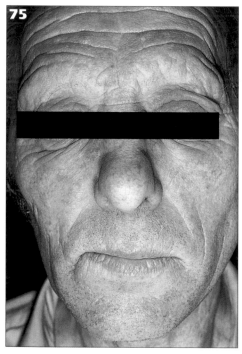

75 Airborne dermatitis caused by dust contaminated with antibiotics.

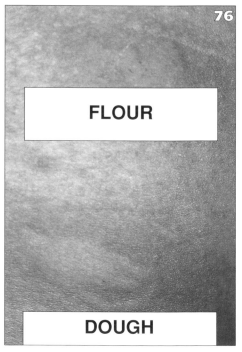

FLOUR

DOUGH

76 A positive scratch-chamber test after using the baker's own flour and dough.

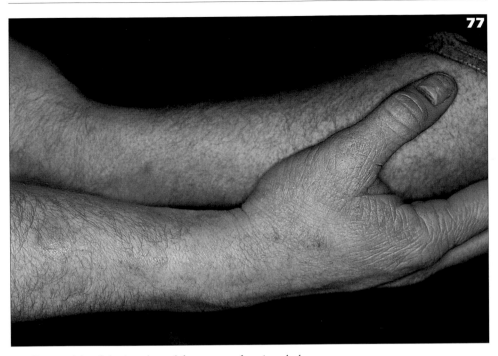

77 Dermatitis of the hands and forearms of a pizza baker.

MANAGEMENT

The rational management of occupational allergic contact dermatitis calls for the correct identification of its cause and the removal of the hapten from the workplace of the patient. In some cases it is possible to exchange the hapten with a non-sensitising substitute. If no substitute can be found an attempt may be made to relocate the sensitised person within the workplace, though this is rarely possible in small businesses or during periods of unemployment. It is also important to provide sufficient information to ensure that the patient can avoid contact with the hapten during non-working hours.

Protective clothing and special training in allergen avoidance has been used as a preventive measure when dealing with epoxy sensitisation. One important means of preventing allergic contact dermatitis in the workplace is the confinement of processes involving sensitisers. This approach is reasonable when dealing with rare or unusual allergens but is, of course, not feasible when the dermatitis is caused by a ubiquitous allergen.

Good personal hygiene and the use of suitable gloves can prevent allergic contact dermatitis in some situations. It should be remembered that gloves are made of a wide variety of materials and that low molecular compounds can penetrate latex gloves. The insides of gloves

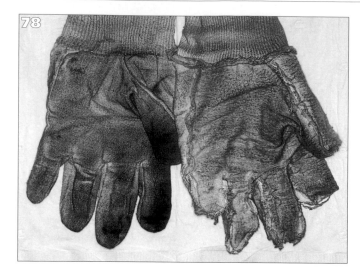

78 (Left) The outside of an originally white protective glove. (Right) The inside of the same glove.

are easily contaminated (**78**) and the use of contaminated gloves can cause aggravation of the dermatitis. Generally speaking, barrier creams are of little use in controlling allergic contact dermatitis. It may be necessary for persons suspected of having allergic contact dermatitis to take sick leave while the cause is determined. However, prolonged absence from the workplace increases the risk of permanent disability. The specific dermato

logical treatment of allergic contact dermatitis does not differ from the treatment of other types of contact dermatitis.

BIBLIOGRAPHY

Cronin, E (1980), *Contact Dermatitis*, Churchill Livingstone, Edinburgh.
Veien, NK (1995), Clinical features, *Textbook of Contact Dermatitis*, Springer-Verlag, Berlin, 153–204.

CHAPTER FOUR

OCCUPATIONAL SKIN DISORDERS ASSOCIATED WITH SUN OR ARTIFICIAL LIGHT EXPOSURE

James Ferguson

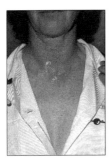

UVB burns can occur from therapy units.

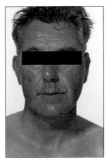

Drug-induced phototoxicity.

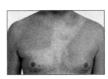

Solar urticaria.

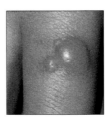

Psoralen-induced phototoxicity.

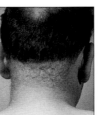

Phenothiazine-induced photoallergic contact dermatitis.

INTRODUCTION

Providing that UVB (280–320 nm) or the shorter wavelengths of UVA (320–340 nm) are present in adequate amounts, exposure of the normal skin will show acute and chronic effects (*Table 10*). While all humans have the potential for such responses, some particularly susceptible individuals with fair skin will show such effects with much lower exposures.

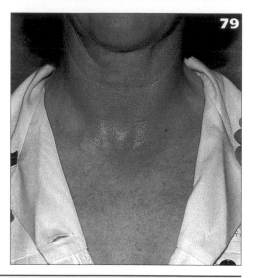

79 Acute sunburn in a hospital technician accidentally exposed to excessive UVB from a therapy unit.

Table 10. Acute and chronic ultraviolet effects in the normal population.

Ultraviolet effects	Clinical features
Acute	
Sunburn	Erythema (**79**)
	Pain/swelling
	Blistering
Welder's flash (photokeratitis)	Corneal pain/scarring
Provocation of cold sores	Vesiculation, usually face (**80**)
Chronic	
Ageing	Wrinkles
	Dryness
	Laxity (**81, 82**)
Photocarcinogenesis	Tumours

NORMAL REACTIONS

Disorders are subdivided into those that affect the normal population (*Table 10*) and those with a pre-existing photosensitivity disorder or abnormal susceptibility.

Outdoor occupations associated with extensive ultraviolet exposure are traditionally farming, market gardening, forestry, working on the road and build-ing. Such workers may be exposed to excessive sunlight. Those who have artificial ultraviolet sources in their workplace include welders, industrial manufacture workers using certain processes, university researchers, hospital technicians and nurses, shopkeepers and sunbed parlour operators (*Tables 11, 12*).

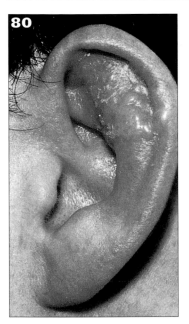

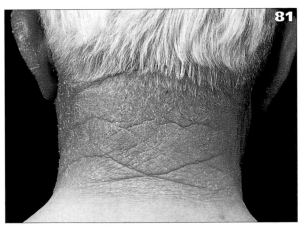

81 Severe elastotic change on the back of the neck in a farmer (cutis rhomboidalis nuchae).

80 A herpes simplex lesion (cold sore) activated in a medical physics technician who had experienced acute sunburn one week previously after accidental UVB exposure.

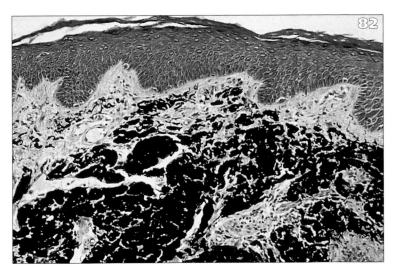

82 Histology (Elastica stain) reveals marked dermal solar elastosis.

Table 11. Environmental ultraviolet sources.

Source	Wavelengths	Occupation
Natural		
Sunlight (at the surface of of the Earth)	UVB/A	Outdoor workers
Artificial		
Electric arc welding	UVC/B/A	Welders and co-workers
Sunbeds/recreational sources	UVA/B	Solarium staff
UV industrial/research lamps	UVB/A	Industry Printers Research workers
Bacteriocidal lamps	UVC/B/A	Research workers
Phototherapy units	UVB/A	Health care workers Nurses/technicians

Table 12. Annual, unintentional, natural ultraviolet exposures of indoor and outdoor workers in mid-latitudes (40°–60°N).

Worker	UVB (MED)	UVA (J/cm^2)
Outdoor	250	3000
Indoor	70	1000

MED = Minimal erythema dose

PHOTOTOXICITY

Exposure to a photosensitiser may make a normal subject artificially susceptible to ultraviolet visible irradiation. A phototoxic reaction will occur in the majority of subjects provided that enough chemical and irradiation of appropriate wavelength are present. Examples of phototoxic agents (systemic and contact) are listed in *Table 13*; some photosensitisers are associated with particular occupations.

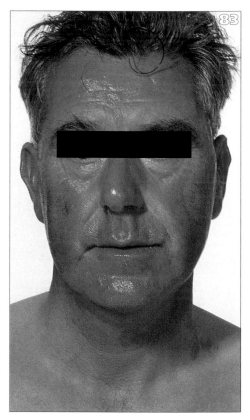

83 Amiodarone phototoxicity induced 'golden brown' pigmentation in a gardener.

Table 13. Examples of known phototoxic agents which will potentially produce skin reactions in the normal population.

Agent	Occupations at particular risk
Systemic	All high UV exposure groups
Thiazides	
Amiodarone (**83**)	
Chlorpromazine	
Non-steroidal anti-inflammatories	
Antibiotics	
Quinine (**84**)	
Topical	
Coal tars and related agents	Tar distillers; road labourers
Phytophotodermatitis (see Chapter 7)	
Psoralens:	Farm workers; canning
celery (particularly if infected with pink rot)	workers; cooks (**85**)
parsnips	
figs	
Umbelliferae weeds (strimmer's dermatitis)	Farm/estate workers (**86, 87**)
Drugs:	Pharmaceutical workers; human
chlorpromazine	and animal care workers
Dyestuffs:	
benzanthrone	Manufacture process workers (**88**)
disperse blue 35	Ultraviolet curing ink workers
amyldismethylaminobenzoate	

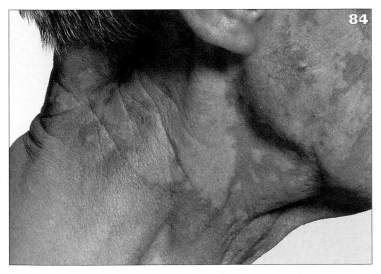

84 Quinine-induced photoleucomelanoderma in a road inspector.

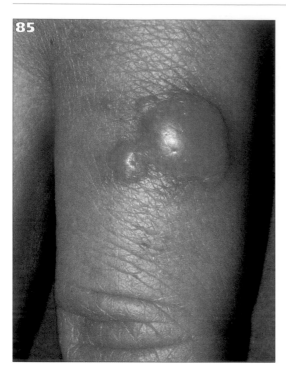

85 After making a large batch of celery soup this patient used a sunbed producing phototoxic blisters 48 hours later on the backs of her hands.

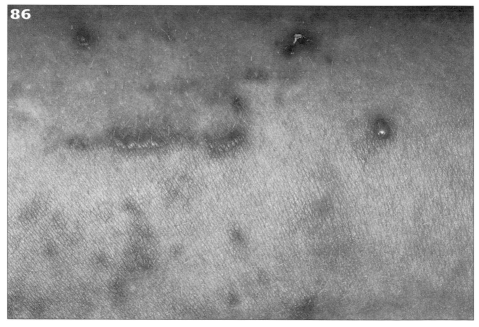

86 Linear erythema and blisters arising 48 hours after using a strimmer on a summer's day (psoralen phytophotodermatitis).

87 Persistent pigmentation (melanin) 3 weeks following strimmer's phytophotodermatitis.

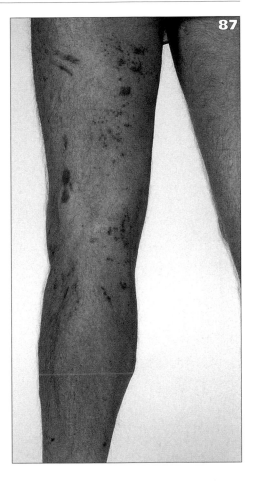

88 Painful phototoxic erythema and swelling followed sunlight exposure in this benzanthrone manufacturing worker.

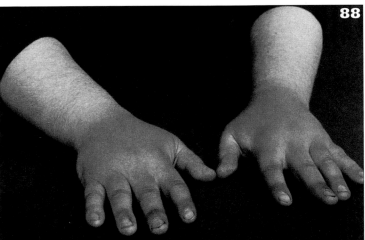

PHOTOALLERGY

Photoallergy is an uncommon skin reaction to light and photosensitiser in which a sensitised immune process is involved (this is considered under the abnormal response group).

Abnormal reactions

A more susceptible group are those affected by the photosensitive diseases (*Table 14*).

THE IDIOPATHIC PHOTO-DERMATOSES

Severe abnormal photosensitivity may be a feature of this group of conditions. Photosensitivity dermatitis/actinic reticuloid syndrome (PD/AR)/chronic actinic dermatitis photosensitivity frequently extends into the visible waveband region with skin reactions which may follow exposure to as little as 1/100 of the radiation dose required to induce an erythema response in normal individuals. Even indoor occupations may prove difficult for these patients. The associated abnormality of multiple contact allergy is another important reason for continuing problems at work seen here in a market gardener (**89**) and an estate worker (**90**).

Polymorphic light eruption (PLE), although usually less severe than PD/AR, may cause occupational problems, with as little as 5 minutes of outdoor sunlight or sunlight transmitted through window-glass capable of inducing the problem

Table 14. Photosensitive diseases.

Idiopathic photodermatoses

Photosensitivity dermatitis/actinic reticuloid syndrome (PD/AR) (chronic actinic dermatitis)
Multiple contact allergy to plants and other agents (**89, 90**)
Solar urticaria (SU) (**92**)
Hydroa vacciniforme (HV)
Polymorphic light eruption (PLE) (**91**)

Photocontact reactions

Phototoxicity (see also *Tables 11, 12*)
Photoallergy:
  halogenated salicylanilides (**93**)
  quindoxin
  chlorpromazine (**94**)
  fragrances
  sunscreens

Genophotodermatoses

Porphyrias

Photoaggravated disorders

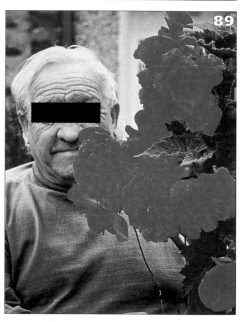

89 Market gardener with PD/AR syndrome known to have plant contact allergy.

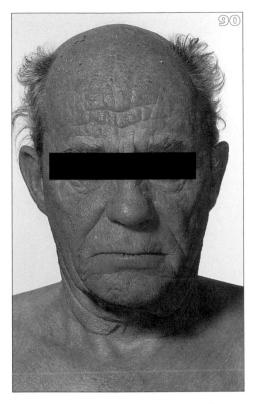

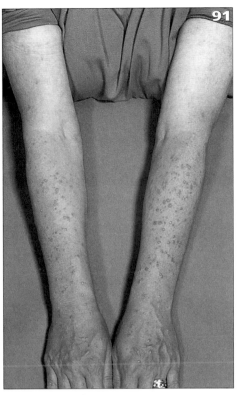

90 Forestry worker with PD/AR syndrome and known sensitivity to usnic acid.

91 Municipal garden worker with work-related, sunlight-induced PLE.

92 Solar urticaria, induced by visible wavelengths, in a chauffeur. Note the area protected by the seat-belt

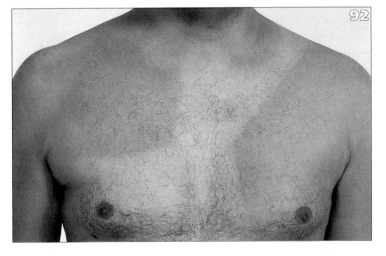

(**91**). Solar urticaria sensitivity frequently extends into the visible wavelength region and may necessitate a change of occupation (**92**).

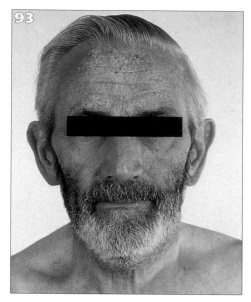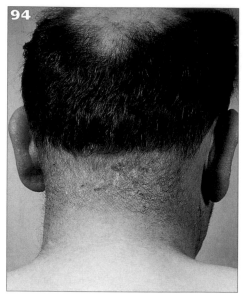

93 Photoallergy in a factory worker who worked with soap containing tetrachlorosalicylaniside.

94 Health care worker who developed chlorpromazine-induced photoallergy after crushing tablets to enable a patient to swallow medicine.

Photoallergy of a photocontact type is a rare event although reported with a range of occupational chemicals (93, 94). In general, when these chemicals are recognised, they then tend to be replaced by non-photoallergenic alternatives.

at particular risk due to abnormal photosensitivity will allow prevention of the disorder by controlling exposure to it. Usual measures include a change of environment and the use of clothing and sunscreening with topical agents.

MANAGEMENT

Awareness of exposure to occupational UV and visible wavelength light, of potential photosensitisers and of those subjects

BIBLIOGRAPHY

Diffey, BL (1992), Human exposure to ultraviolet radiation, *The Environmental Threat to the Skin*, Martin Dunitz, London, 3–9.

CHAPTER FIVE

MISCELLANEOUS OCCUPATIONAL DERMATOSES

Michael H Beck and John SC English

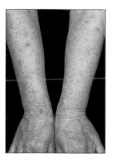

The dermatitis looked irritant, but the patient was allergic to an epoxy compound in machining oil.

Vesicular palmar eczema was not endogenous, but an allergy that resulted from IPPD.

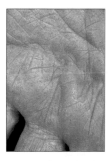

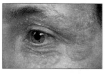

Atopic eczema aggravated by allergic contact dermatitis.

Pulpitis due to irritant contact dermatitis.

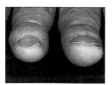

Methacrylate sealants can cause onycholysis and dermatitis.

Cold urticaria from handling cold clay.

INTRODUCTION

In this chapter various examples of contact dermatitis and other work-related dermatoses not covered elsewhere in the book are illustrated.

DERMATITIS

Figures **95–128** provide a comprehensive picture gallery of various types of dermatitis.

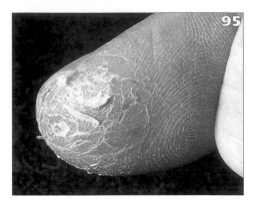

95 Chromate exposure may be difficult to pinpoint. The health and safety data sheets confirmed hexavalent chromate to be in the sealant which came into contact with the tips of this aircraft construction worker's thumb, forefinger and middle finger when dipping rivets into it.

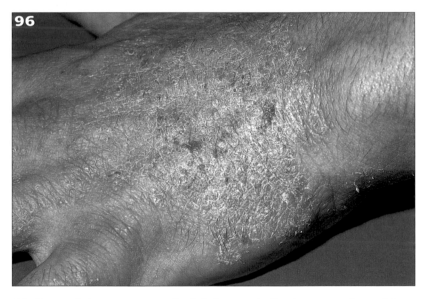

96 Cement is known to cause both irritant and allergic contact dermatitis. The latter is from the chromate content. Chromate allergy from this source may induce a discoid pattern of eczema which can be confused with constitutional eczema. The dermatitis may persist despite changing occupation. 'Hardening' often develops so that the individual can stay at work without severe disability.

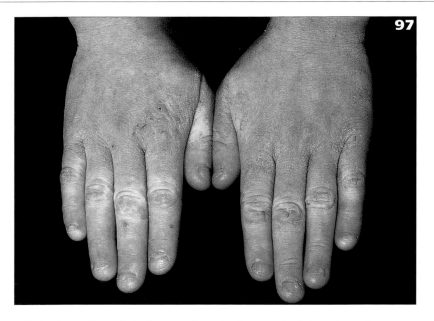

97 Coolant oils used during metal machining may be irritant but also contain allergens. Irritant contact dermatitis, as shown here, appears to be less frequent than formerly because of the increased automation of metal working machines. Usually protective gloves are not used with moving machinery parts for safety reasons.

98 This woman worked with a cutting oil; her pattern is that of an irritant contact dermatitis. However, patch testing revealed that she was allergic to epoxy resin and to the oil. The ingredient that caused the cross-reaction with epoxy resin was 1,2-cyclohexane dicarboxylic acid, bis(oxyrinylmethyl) ester. It is an epoxy compound containing two epoxide groups and was used as a chlorine ion scavenger in the oil.

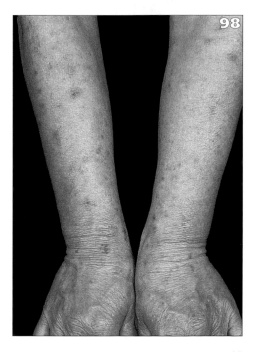

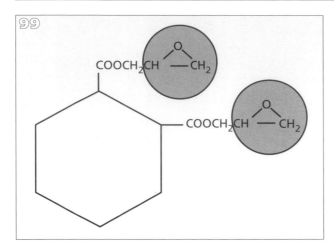

99 1,2-cyclohexane dicarboxylic acid, bis(oxyrinylmethyl) ester, or diglycidyl ester of hexahydrophthalic acid. The epoxy groups are shaded.

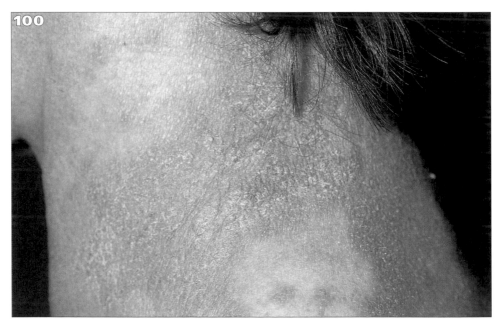

100 Epoxy resins when uncured, and the hardeners themselves, may induce contact allergy. The skin affected often involves all the exposed sites as epoxy resin oligomers become volatile during the exothermic hardening process. This individual was spraying a 'two part' paint.

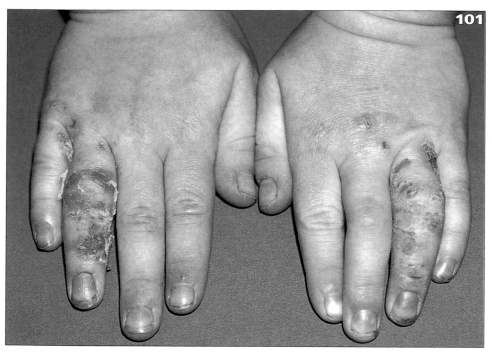

101 This publican developed an acute irritant contact dermatitis after his hands were in contact with acid cleanser used to clean out pipes in his pub.

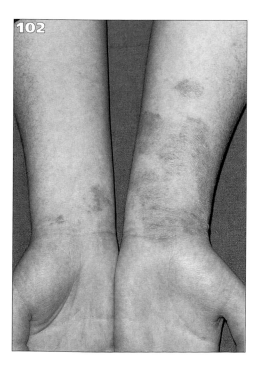

102 Irritant contact dermatitis is common amongst those undertaking cleaning and washing duties. This restaurant worker found that detergent and water gained access through the open ends of her gloves. The gloves then occlude the irritant materials, exacerbating the situation.

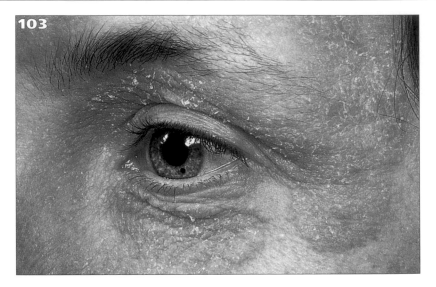

103 Patch testing is an important investigation for individuals with flares of chronic eczematous eruptions. This woman was thought to have an exacerbation of her well-established atopic eczema. She was allergic to colophony released by solder fumes in the factory where she gave out worksheets Her acute facial rash settled down on removal from this working environment.

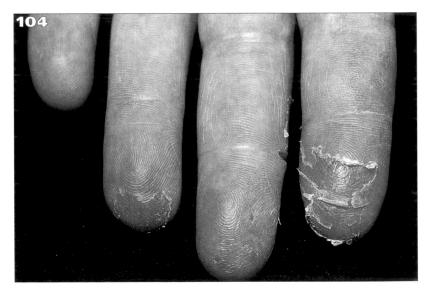

104 This dentist had a fissuring skin eruption involving the finger tips, particularly of the fore-, middle and ring fingers of the dominant hand. He was allergic to a number of acrylic monomers used in the UV-cured fillings. Acrylic monomers can cause dermatitis from many other occupational sources, most notably in locking glues (Locktite™), UV-cured printing plates and denture manufacture.

105 This foundry worker had a low grade irritation and erythema of his hands. He was in contact with resinated sand used to make moulds. He was allergic to the phenol formaldehyde resin used in the sand, but not to the phenol formaldehyde resin from a plastic series. Phenol formaldehyde resins' allergenicity vary according to the source. It is important to patch test with the type of phenol formaldehyde resin actually used by the patient.

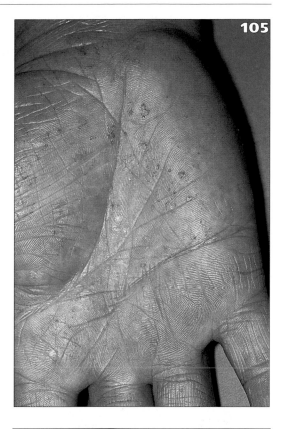

106 Textile dermatitis is usually caused by formaldehyde and formaldehyde resins found particularly in cotton clothing and also from dyes in nylon clothing. The distribution around rather than within the body folds is typical. In this instance the cause was allergy to disperse nylon dyes in this airline pilot's uniform.

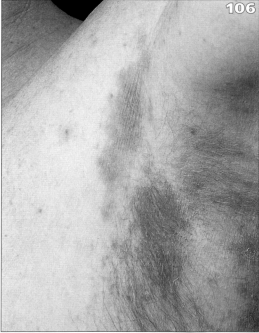

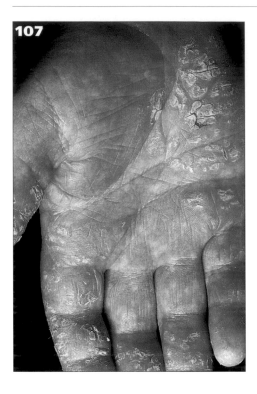

107 This man's hand eruption looks distinctly psoriasiform. He was shown to be allergic to thiuram which is used as an accelerator in the manufacture of rubber. He settled with treatment after redeployment away from contact with rubber components in his work.

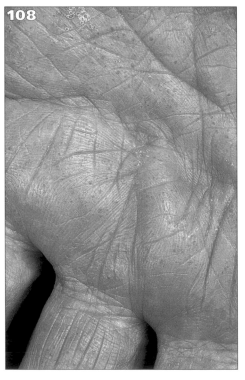

108 Allergic contact dermatitis from isopropyl phenyl-*p*-phenylenediamine (IPPD) can cause a very chronic endogenous-looking vesicular palmar hand dermatitis. This man worked in tyre manufacturing.

109 This man performed clerical work and was only diagnosed as having occupational dermatitis after patch tests. His skin disorder followed a palmar distribution, particularly on the non-dominant hand. He was shown to be allergic to IPPD. He worked for the Police Forensic Department taking down details of car tyre treads which he would handle!

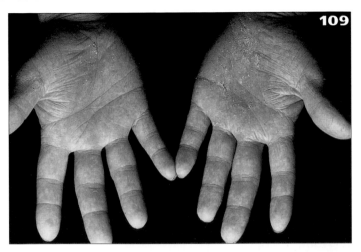

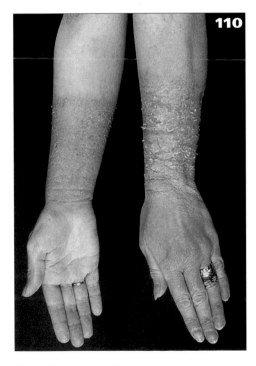

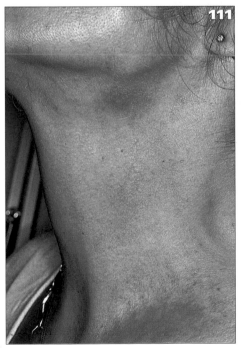

110 Allergy to rubber in gloves and footwear should always be considered as a possibility in persistent rashes of the hands and feet. Not all cases are as obvious as this one. The allergens are usually anti-oxidants or accelerators in the rubber.

111 Dermatitis and acneiform skin eruptions can result from frictional trauma. An example is shown here in a professional violinist caused by her chin rest. This is known as 'fiddler's neck' (see Chapter 7).

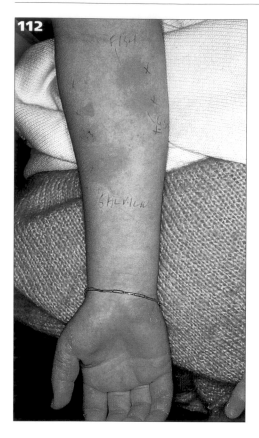

112 Contact allergy of the immediate and delayed type was first noted in Danish sandwich makers. It is shown here in a chef with hand eczema with positive prick tests on the forearm to cod and prawn (see Chapter 3).

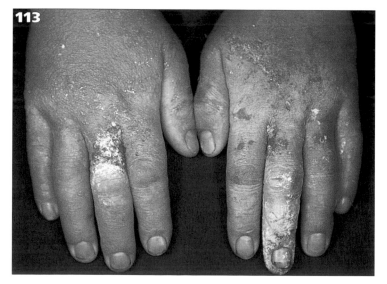

113 Food handlers are particularly prone to irritant contact dermatitis from raw meat, fish, fruit and vegetable juices. This man had negative patch and prick tests.

114 Trauma, particularly from friction, is a commonly overlooked source for dermatitis. This market trader spent much of the day loading and unloading suitcases, causing a frictional dermatitis consisting of erythema, scaling and fissuring predominantly on his dominant right palm.

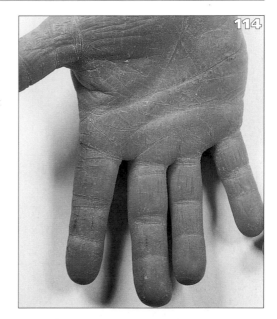

115 Hairdressers are a group especially prone to irritant and allergic contact dermatitis from the chemicals used in the salon. Glyceryl monothioglycolate used in 'acid' perms is a frequent allergen. Its allergenicity persists in the hair and stylists may have significant dermatitis between the fingers of their non-dominant hand as a result of holding the hair whilst cutting it.

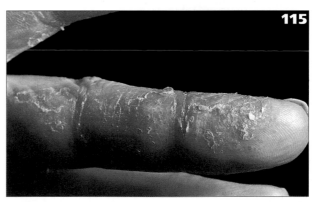

116 This woman's unprotected hands were in contact with shampoo and bubble bath materials whilst filling bottles. She has developed an irritant contact dermatitis and her allergy to Kathon CG (5-chloro-2-methyl-4-isothiazolin-3-one) used as a biocide in the products may have been a secondary event.

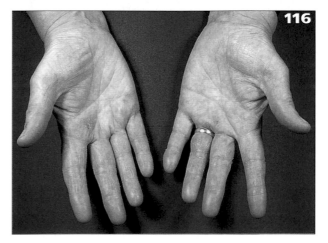

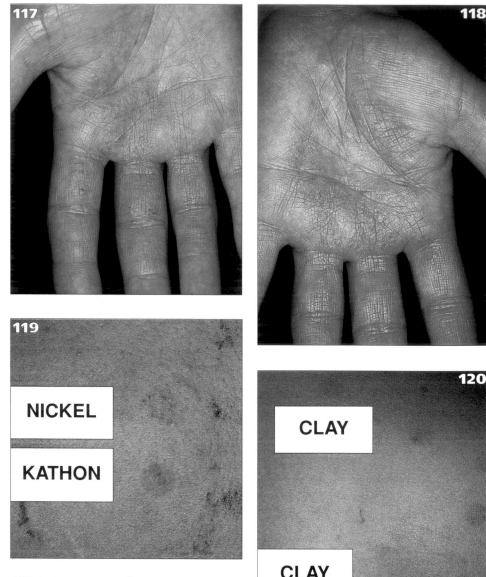

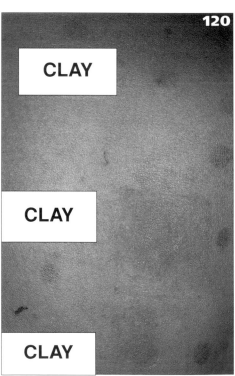

117, 118, 119, 120 This woman modelled flowers out of clay. She would roll the clay in the palm of her left hand with the ball of her right hand. Up until 2 years prior to presentation she had never had any trouble. Then a biocide was added to the clay and after a few months she developed dermatitis. Patch tests revealed positives to nickel, Kathon CG and to the clay (as is). The biocide was removed from the clay and her dermatitis completely cleared.

121, 122 This patient applied transfers to pottery ware as a lithographer. It involved slipping the transfers off when wet and using a rubber sponge to squeeze out any bubbles from under the transfers on the plate. Her right hand would be in contact with water and a detergent for the greater part of the working day, hence she developed irritant contact dermatitis on her thumb, second and third fingers. This is a common pattern in lithographers in the pottery industry.

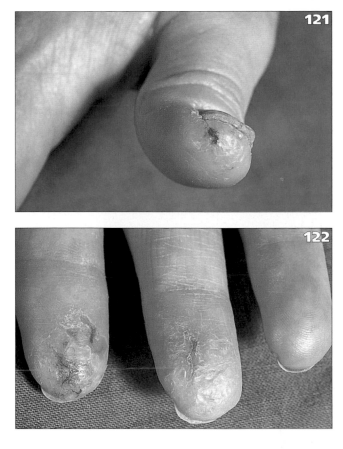

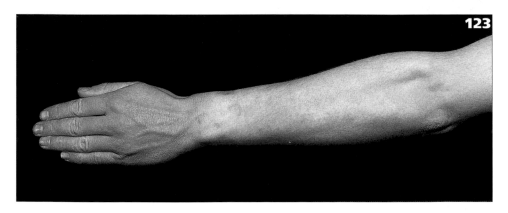

123 This man handled blueprints in an architect's office. He developed a photo-allergy to thiourea used in the paper and his photosensitivity was noted to continue despite avoidance. This is a recognised phenomenon known as persistent light reaction.

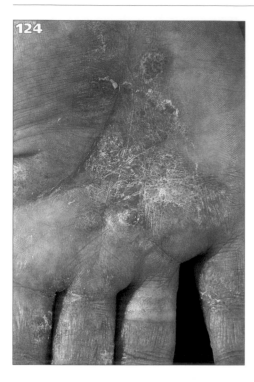

124 Nickel sensitisation affects at least 10% of the female population. Subsequent development of hand eczema in affected subjects often carries a poor prognosis. Allergy commonly develops following ear piercing and can present with a skin eruption under nickel-containing clothing components and jewellery when there is close contact. In this patient, however, primary sensitisation occurred from contact with traumatising tiny metal fragments encountered in her work as a key cutter.

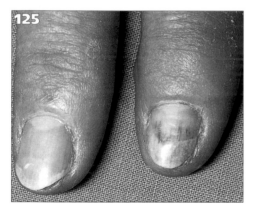

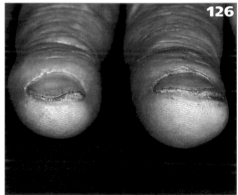

125 Beauticians and nail technicians may handle acrylic monomers when making sculptured nails. Allergy will cause a contact dermatitis. Often the beauticians will wear this form of nail themselves. They are produced by mixing a powder and liquid. Painful onycholysis has resulted in this sensitised beautician wearing such nails.

126 This man has allergic contact dermatitis from Loctite™ sealant. He had a positive patch test to ethylene glycol dimethacrylate.

127 Minor injuries at work may require a visit to the First Aid department. Many creams used on cuts and abrasions contain contact sensitisers, e.g. topical anaesthetics and antihistamines. This appearance was caused by a benzocaine-containing cream applied to an abrasion.

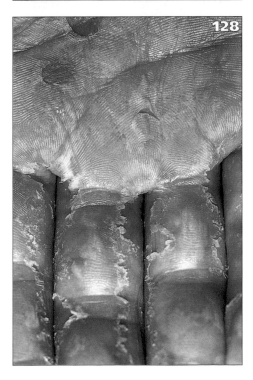

128 Acute chemical burn with sloughing of the superficial layers of the skin after inadvertent contact with trisodium phosphate.

URTICARIA

Figures **129** and **130** demonstrate occupational physical urticaria.

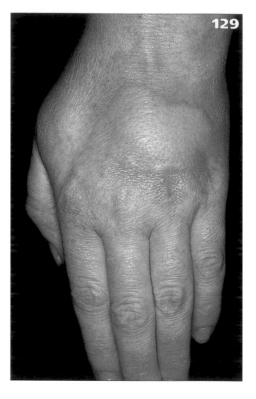

129 This patient had cold urticaria. When she handled cold, wet clay she would develop urticarial lesions on her hands. She did not suffer quite so badly in the summer.

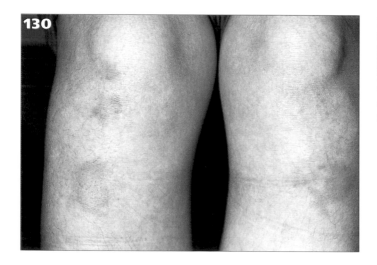

130 This woman suffered from delayed pressure urticaria. Her job as a cleaner involved kneeling at work, and she would develop lesions at the end of the day's work.

MISCELLANEOUS

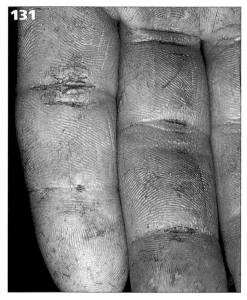

Finally, **131–137** illustrate various other forms of occupational dermatoses.

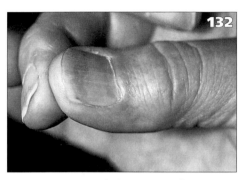

132 Pressure onycholysis in a tailor, caused by holding his needle.

131 This slaughterhouse worker developed a painful callus on his second finger, caused by friction from the handle of his knife.

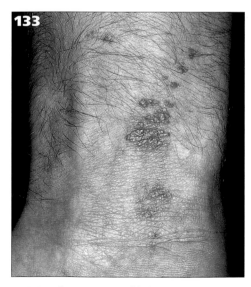

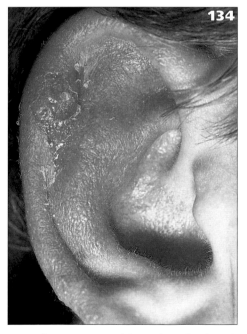

133 Koebnerisation of lichen planus on a forklift truck driver's wrist. He had to hold heavy ropes away from the truck, which would drag on the inside of his right wrist.

134 This newspaper delivery boy developed frost-bite, one cold winter, on his ears. He wore a baseball cap; a woolly hat to cover his ears would have been better.

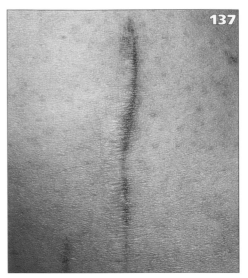

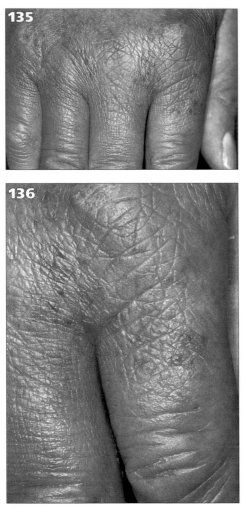

137 This elderly coal miner had a coal tattoo on his shoulder. Scrapes in underground workers on the skin and coal tattooing is very common.

135, 136 Pieces of rock embedded in the skin of a stonemason. This is effectively tattooing of the skin.

BIBLIOGRAPHY

Adams, RM (1990), *Occupational Skin Disease*, W.B. Saunders Co., Philadelphia.

CHAPTER SIX

DIFFERENTIAL DIAGNOSIS OF HAND ECZEMA

Henk B van der Walle

Unilateral palmar scaling usually means fungus infection.

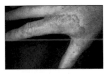

Sharp demarcation and active edge are diagnostic of fungus infection.

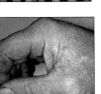

Chronic irritant contact dermatitis is diagnosed by occupation, clinical pattern and negative patch tests.

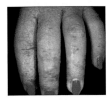

Allergic contact dermatitis is diagnosed by occupation, clinical pattern and a positive patch test.

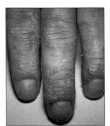

Atopic hand eczema is a risk factor for developing irritant contact dermatitis.

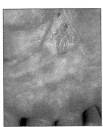

Palmar psoriasis tends to be dry and scaly, with painful fissures; the dermatitis is usually very itchy.

INTRODUCTION

The hands are important organs for communication and manipulation. Hand eczema impairs the work capability and social intercourse of patients and affects their economical and psychosocial stability. The name 'eczema' embraces a variety of skin disorders with different origins and patterns; the course, treatment and prognosis strongly depend on the cause of the eczema. Therefore the diagnosis is the starting point for the management and treatment of the individual patient.

DIAGNOSIS

The diagnosis is the outcome of a process of collecting and interpreting facts. These facts are derived from clinical inspection, history, microscopy, bacterial culture, patch testing, histopathology and workplace inspection. Sometimes a definite diagnosis can be made just with a glance but additional investigations are often necessary.

The clinical picture holds important keys to the diagnosis, and attention should be focused on localisation, demarcation and morphological features such as redness, vesicles, blisters, necrosis, papules, scaling, fissures, infections or eczema. Besides the lesions on the hands, other skin parts should be examined, with special attention to the skin of the face, neck and feet. The patient should be screened for symptoms of atopic dermatitis, psoriasis or active eczema.

Hand eczema may have a course with improvements and exacerbations, implying that the dermatologist is often not confronted with a dermatitis in the active phase. Sometimes it is necessary to request the patient to return with a relapse of the eczema.

Questioning of the patient is guided by the characteristics of the clinical picture and his or her daily activities. An extensive history of the patient's activities at work, in hobbies and at home is essential, with special attention to the materials and tools handled. Sometimes it is necessary to visit the workplace or consult the occupational hygienist to obtain a good impression of the exposure in the occupation. Attention should be paid to the use of gloves, skin care products and medication.

The course of the dermatitis may offer important keys to the final diagnosis. Relationships must be checked between improvements and relapses of the dermatitis and activities in occupation, the home environment, weekends, holidays, sick leave and the use of gloves.

Patch testing is obligatory in nearly all cases of hand eczema. This testing should focus on exposure to allergens in occupation, home environment, skin-care products and cosmetics; in many cases a combination of diagnoses will be made. The most common diagnoses are allergic contact dermatitis, cumulative irritant contact dermatitis, atopic dermatitis and psoriasis. The different diagnoses described in the following section are those commonly stated in the literature. These categories are not absolute – some may overlap and others will be redefined or disappear in the future based on any advance in our knowledge.

DIFFERENTIAL DIAGNOSIS

Fungus infection

In general two patterns of infection can be observed. First, there is a dry, scaly dermatitis with a slight redness on the palms and the palmar aspect of the fingers, and often combined with ony-chomycosis; no involvement of wrist or forearm, and almost exclusively unilateral. The second pattern (also unilateral) occurs on the dorsum of the hand and fingers, with scattered papules, vesicles or pustules, or with a ring-type dermatitis with an active edge and scaling. Onychomycosis may occur. Both patterns may be altered by the use of topical corticosteroids (**138–141**).

Key to diagnosis

Unilateral localisation; positive KOH microscopy; onychomycosis.

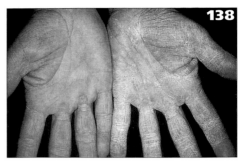

138 Fungus infection of the left hand with typical unilateral localisation.

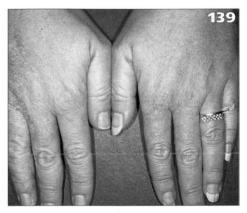

139 Contact dermatitis can be unilateral as in this right-handed hairdresser with allergic contact dermatitis from glyceryl monothioglycolate. Skin scrapings for mycological examination should be taken if diagnosis is in doubt.

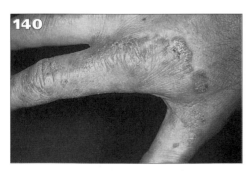

140 Fungus infection with sharp demarcation.

141 Compare **140** with this sharply demarcated cumulative irritant contact dermatitis in a cleaner with a history of childhood atopic dermatitis.

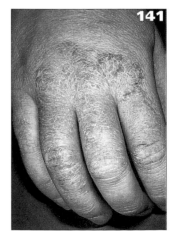

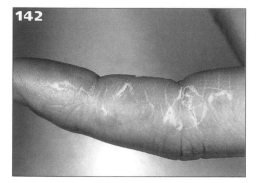

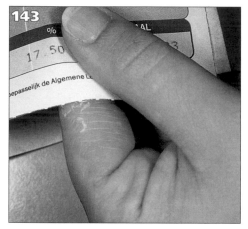

142, 143 'Mechanical' dermatitis, induced by the daily manipulation of paperwork in a bank employee.

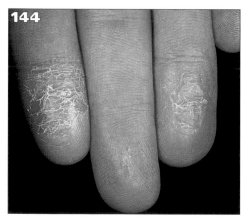

144 Fingertip dermatitis, induced by manipulating rough paper in a patient with psoriasis.

Mechanical trauma

Skin disorders caused by mechanical injury develop at the site of the injury. Friction, pressure and shearing forces may cause dermatitis, hyperkeratosis, callosities, corns, blisters and abrasions. Handling dry and rough materials may induce a circumscribed dermatitis with a dry, scaly appearance which mimics psoriasis. This occurs exclusively on the distal and palmar side of one or two fingers; there is no nail involvement (142–145).

Key to diagnosis

Evaluation of exposure.

Cumulative irritant contact dermatitis

This is caused by the repetition of the same damaging factor or the cumulative effect of a variety of minor damaging factors (see Chapter 2). In many wet-work occupations the clinically normal skin is damaged on a sub-clinical level by exposure to water, soap and detergents. A slight erythema with fine scaling is the first visible sign of damage. A sudden change in occupational exposure or in climate conditions may push the damage from this sub-clinical level 'over the edge' to a clearly visible contact dermatitis with redness, oedema, scaling, chapping (i.e. fissures in the horny layer), erythema craquelé (i.e. fissures going deeper into the epidermis) or even to haemorrhagic fissures caused by cracks reaching into the dermis.

In longstanding cases the clinical picture may vary from a dry palmar dermatitis with erythema, fine scaling, chapping and shiny fingertips (in so-called wear and tear dermatitis as seen in

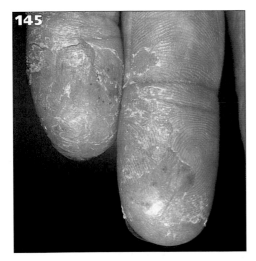

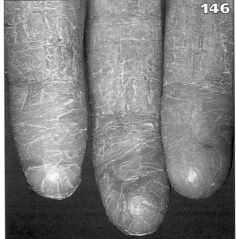

145 Allergic contact dermatitis, due to acrylic monomer, on the fingertips of a printer. The presence of healing vesicles makes a dermatitis more likely than psoriasis.

146 Cumulative irritant contact dermatitis in housewife with four small children. Dermatitis is usually itchy whereas psoriasis is usually dry, scaly and the skin splits – which is sore – and bleeds.

cleaning and housekeeping) to a more eczematous dermatitis with itch, erythema, oedema and lichenification. Any part of the hands may be involved, but there are general characteristics. Chapping is predominantly seen on the back of the hands while fissures and cracks are seen on the dorsal bending parts of the fingers and in the palm (**146, 147**).

Fissures and cracks at the fingertips often occur in occupations such as painting and printing with prolonged exposure to organic solvents. Finger web dermatitis occurs in wet-work occupations and may spread to the back of the hands. The localisation of contact dermatitis may be determined by the use of the right or left hand in certain occupations – if the dominant hand is exposed to the irritant, the dermatitis will occur on this hand, but in many occupations the dominant hand is used for handling tools or instruments and the non-dominant hand is exposed to water and other irritants. The nail may

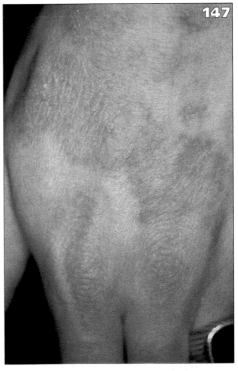

147 Cumulative irritant contact dermatitis with patchy distribution in a hairdresser.

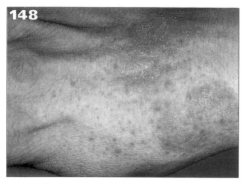

show onycholysis, sub-ungual hyperkeratosis, textural irregularities of the nail with pitting and transverse depressions. Nail folds may become red and swollen, with painful fissures at the transition with the nail (148–152).

Key to diagnosis

Occupation; localisation; negative patch test.

148 Allergic contact dermatitis in a nurse, due to thiuram compound in gloves. The clinical appearance does not always give the correct diagnosis unless the patient is patch tested.

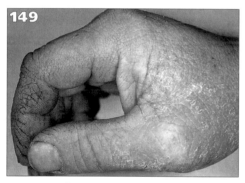

149 Cumulative chronic irritant contact dermatitis in a car mechanic.

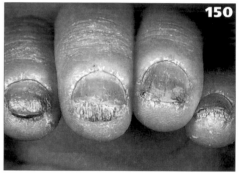

150 Cumulative irritant contact dermatitis of the nail and nail folds in a car mechanic.

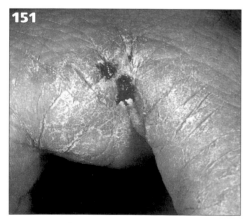

151 Cumulative irritant contact dermatitis with painful fissures.

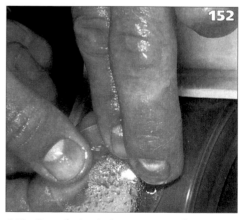

152 Cumulative irritant contact dermatitis on a fingertip in an optician, caused by a water jet during glass cutting.

Allergic contact dermatitis

Type 4 hypersensitivity reactions can induce skin disorders with many different clinical pictures. The spectrum varies from pompholyx-like vesicles on one finger, a fingertip dermatitis on the serving hand and streaks of sharply demarcated erythema on the dorsum of the hand, to a very active eczema of both hands with marked oedema and total impairment of hand functions. Secondary spread to the face, neck, axillae and genitals frequently occurs. Itch is a dominating factor; the typical course is with improvements and exacerbations.

The chronic forms may continue after stopping contact with the causative allergen(s). A positive patch test is a pre-requisite to establish the diagnosis, but for every positive test the relevance has to be established. Beware of false-negative and false-positive reactions. A positive reaction should never be used to satisfy the doctor's and patient's desire to have a 'cause'. Differentiating allergic contact dermatitis from cumulative irritant contact dermatitis is often a challenge (153–159). *Table 15* summarises important points of difference.

Key to diagnosis

Localisation; occupation; relevant positive patch test.

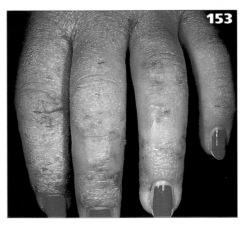

153 Sub-acute allergic contact dermatitis with 'sausage-like' fingers in a hairdresser.

Table 15. Characteristics of cumulative irritant and allergic contact dermatitis.

Characteristic	Cumulative irritant contact dermatitis	Allergic contact dermatitis
Lesions	Oligomorphic with redness, scaling, chapping	Polymorphic with redness, papules, vesicles, crusts, exudation, erosions, lichenification
Demarcation	Patchy, relatively clear	Diffuse; tendency to spread (face, wrist, axillae, genitals)
Localisation	Fingertips, finger webs, dorsum of the hand, ball of the thumb	Interdigital; fingers, palmar and dorsal sides
Course	Chronic; aggravation by climate changes, wet work, detergents, gloves	Relapsing, healing in weekends and holidays
Epidemiology	More persons affected in same work environment	One person affected in same work environment
Patch testing	Negative/positive: not relevant	Relevant positive/negative: allergen missed!

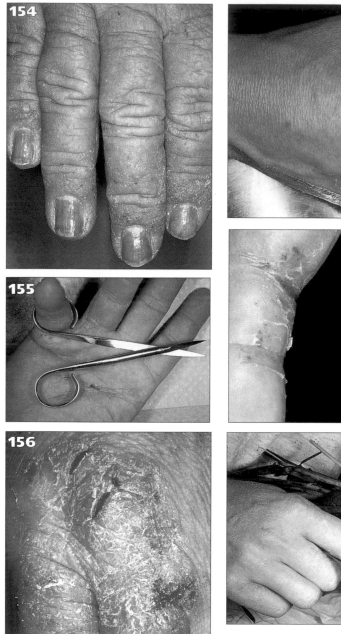

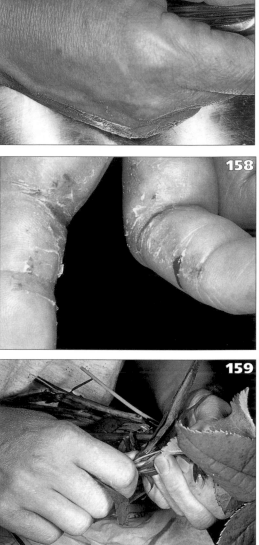

154 Chronic allergic contact dermatitis due to chrysanthemum.

155 Allergic contact dermatitis from nickel due to nickel-releasing scissors of a spinner.

156, 157 A combination of cumulative irritant contact and allergic contact dermatitis from nickel in a hospital employee who exposed the dorsum of his hand to a wet 'stainless' table.

158, 159 Painful allergic contact dermatitis with fissures on the inner sides of the second and third fingers used to strip *Alstroemeria* leaves from the stem.

Atopic dermatitis

The clinical picture of atopic dermatitis is variable and often influenced by exogenous factors. A careful evaluation of the history, irritant, delayed- and immediate-type allergic reactions and secondary infection are important in establishing the full diagnosis. In most cases atopic hand eczema is more or less symmetrically located on the dorsum of the hands, the fingers and often the wrists. Ill-defined patches with erythema, oedema, lichenification and dryness, sometimes with painful fissures on knuckles and wrists, may dominate the picture.

A centrally located patch of dry, lichenified eczema on the palms may also be an expression of atopy. Some patients experience periods of vesicular eruptions on the palms or on the inner sides of the fingers. In youngsters dermatitis of the finger(tips) with erythema, scaling and fissures may mimic psoriasis (160–162).

Key to diagnosis

History and other skin symptoms of atopic constitution.

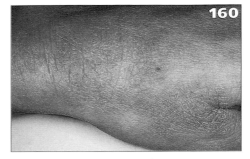

160 Allergic contact dermatitis, due to acrylic monomers, in the owner of a sculptured nail shop.

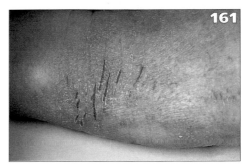

161 Compare 160 with this atopic dermatitis in a housewife with painful fissures at the wrist.

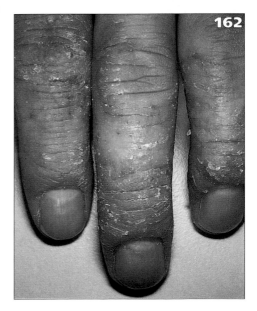

162 A combination of cumulative irritant contact and atopic dermatitis in a male nurse.

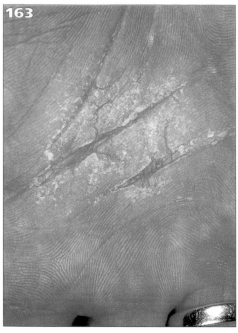

163 Hyperkeratotic dermatitis.

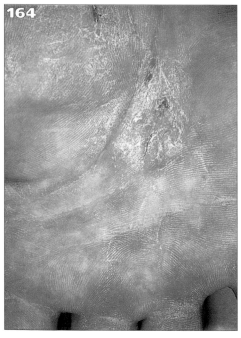

164 Palmar psoriasis with typical extensions to hypothenar prominence. The scaling is more silvery than in hyperkeratotic dermatitis.

Hyperkeratotic dermatitis

Hyperkeratotic dermatitis or tylotic eczema shows hyperkeratotic plaques, centrally located in both palms, with a tendency to painful fissures. The histopathology reveals a slight focal parakeratosis and hyperkeratosis with a spongiotic dermatitis. It is a separate entity which has to be differentiated from psoriasis (*Table 16*, 163, 164).

Key to diagnosis

Circumscribed localisation in the palms; no involvement of other skin parts; no nail changes or signs of arthritis.

Psoriasis

In psoriasis every part of the hand may be affected – nail, fingertips, web areas, palmar and dorsal sides. The clinical picture may vary from a full, red infiltrated skin on the knuckles to a typical psoriatic lesion with redness and yellow waxy scales on a thickened epidermis with an obvious uniformity and well-defined borders. The clinical picture is strongly influenced by exogenous factors, localisation and therapy. Some chronic forms of allergic contact dermatitis may change from an eczematous character into a psoriatic-like lesion (*Table 16*, **165–168**).

Key to diagnosis

Psoriasis on nails and other body parts.

Table 16. Clinical features that help distinguish between palmar psoriasis and hyperkeratotic hand eczema.

Psoriasis	Hyperkeratotic hand eczema
Not usually itchy	Itchy
Painful fissuring	Painful fissuring
Dry, scaly well-defined lesions	Vesicular; scaly
Koebner phenomena	
Nail and knuckle involvement	
More diffuse lesions	

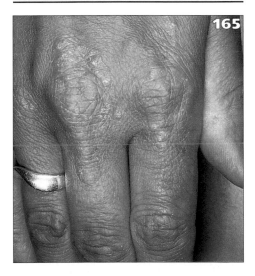

165 Psoriasis on the dorsum of the hands.

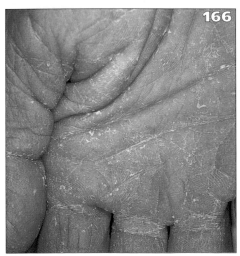

166 Palmar psoriasis in a wet-work occupation.

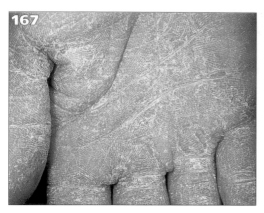

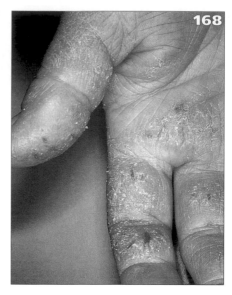

167 Compare **166** with this palmar fungus infection.

168 Compare **166** and **167** with this chronic allergic contact dermatitis in a florist due to handling *Alstroemeria*.

Fingertip eczema

This is a disabling eczema with erythema, scales and painful fissures at the ends of the fingers. Nails may be involved with hyperkeratosis and onycholysis. All fingers may be affected with a preference for the thumb and forefinger of the dominant hand or the fingertips of the serving hand.

Fingertip eczema occurs especially in occupations with such activities as the fine, repetitive handling of food, bulbs, dry materials (including paper) and in professions such as hairdressing and printing. It may be caused by immediate reactions, or by allergic or cumulative irritant contact dermatitis, sometimes in combination with psoriasis and atopic dermatitis (**169–173**).

Key to diagnosis

Localisation; occupation.

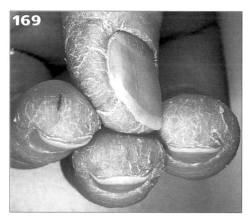

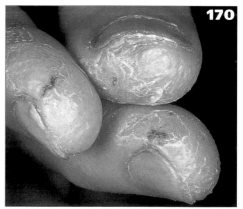

169 Psoriasis on the fingertips.

170 Allergic contact dermatitis with painful fissures in a florist due to handling tulip bulbs.

171 Fingertip psoriasis with sub-ungual hyperkeratosis.

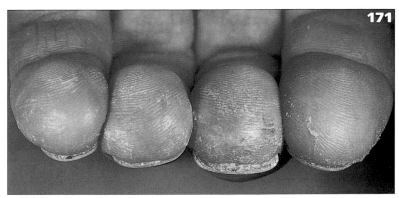

172 Allergic contact dermatitis in a printer, due to acrylic monomer in the printing plates.

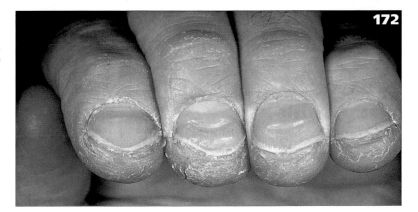

173 Allergic contact dermatitis on the fingertips of a wet hand in a hairdresser with an allergy to glyceryl monothioglycolate.

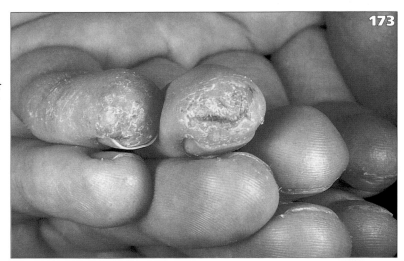

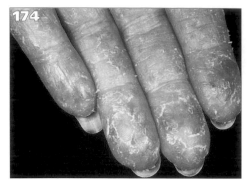

174 Allergic contact dermatitis with lamellar scaling on the palmar side of the hands of a hairdresser due to *p*-phenylene-diamine.

Keratolysis exfoliativa

Keratolysis exfoliativa (or dyshidrosis lamellosa sicca) is the symmetrical occurrence of non-itchy vesicles that dry up and leave typical collarette-type scaling on the palms and the palmar side of the fingers. In some cases there is a typical seasonal variation; this condition may mimic fungus infection. Vesicles in allergic contact dermatitis appear on an inflammatory erythema (**174–176**).

Key to diagnosis

Palmar side of both hands and no erythema.

175 Keratolysis exfoliativa.

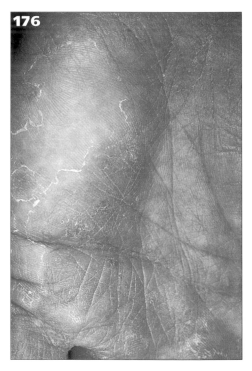

176 Lamellar desquamation in the healing phase of allergic contact dermatitis.

Asteatotic eczema

Asteatotic eczema (or eczema craquelé), which can sometimes be haemorrhagic, shows the aspect of a chapping skin with cracks on a red background; the borders are irregular and slightly raised. Itching is a dominant feature. The preferred localisation is the dorsum of the hands, the upper arms, the lateral sides of the thighs and shins.

In most cases this eczema is a variant of cumulative irritant contact dermatitis with an over-exposure to water (such as in the shower) and soap, especially in winter (**177**).

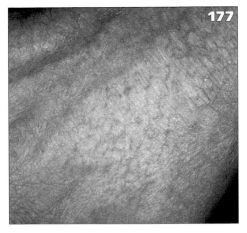

177 Asteatotic eczema (also called eczema craquelé).

Key to diagnosis

Seasonal influence; occupation; craquelé appearance.

Acropustulosis

Acropustulosis (or acrodermatitis perstans) occurs on the distal parts of one or more fingers. It presents as a shiny red, oozing skin with blisters or pustules, with a scaly border of undermined epidermis (**178, 179**).

Key to diagnosis

Sterile culture; localisation.

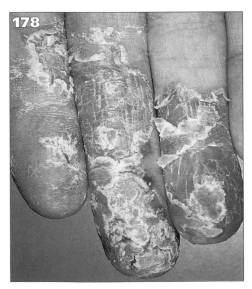

178 Acropustulosis.

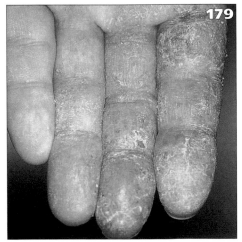

179 Allergic contact dermatitis that mimics acropustulosis in a left-handed person, due to methyldibromoglutaronitril, used as a preservative in a wet wipe.

95

Persistent palmar pustulosis

A shiny red lesion with scales and flat pustules of 1–5 mm diameter. As the pustules dry they change into brown scales. This condition is located centrally in one or both palms and on the thenar and/or hypothenar eminence. A version with red lesions on the heel and sole is common (180, 181).

Key to diagnosis

Sterile culture; lesions on heel or sole; sometimes psoriatic lesions elsewhere.

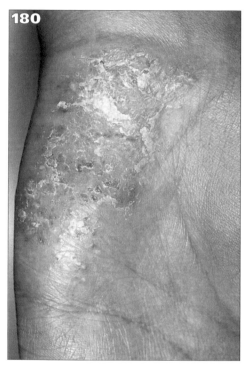

180 Persistent palmar pustulosis.

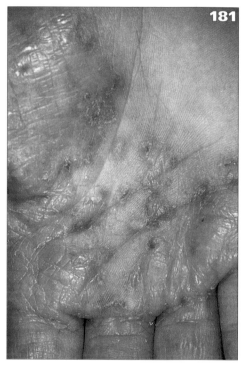

181 Secondarily infected allergic contact dermatitis in a hairdresser.

Secondarily infected dermatitis

Tiny or larger pustules appear in a pre-existing eczema with a preference for the skin between the fingers. There is a sudden aggravation of the eczema with painful redness and oedema, together with general symptoms such as headache and fatigue; sometimes fever may occur. Lymphangitis may be visible on the inner side of the forearm.

Infection often occurs in wet-work professions in combination with cumulative irritant and/or allergic contact dermatitis as in hairdressing,

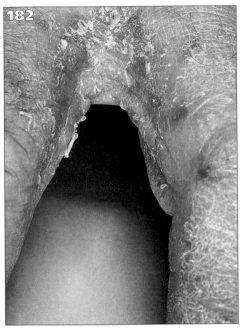

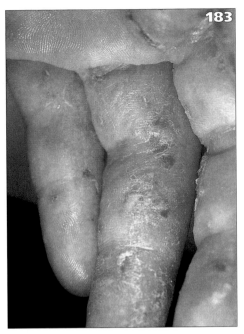

182 Secondarily infected cumulative irritant contact dermatitis in a printer.

183 Allergic contact dermatitis that suddenly worsened due to a secondary infection.

food-handling and hospital work (182, 183).

Key to diagnosis

Rapid deterioration of eczema; general symptoms; positive bacterial culture.

Post-traumatic eczema

Skin injuries caused by abrasions, punctures, or thermal or chemical burns may induce an eczema after an interval of several weeks; it may occur in association with an underlying endogenous eczema. The clinical features are indistinguishable from ordinary eczema. Inspection of the whole body is necessary to detect signs of atopic dermatitis, psoriasis, lichen planus, etc.

Key to diagnosis

Recent trauma.

Post-occupational eczema (persistent occupational dermatitis)

A genuine occupational hand eczema improves when the exposure ceases; relapse or exaggeration occurs by re-exposure. This course, with improvements and exacerbations, may be replaced by a more chronic type of dermatitis, indistinguishable from 'endogenous' eczema, which persists after stopping the exposure. The clinical picture may change from eczematous to a more psoriasiform appearance.

The mechanism and the relation with a 'dormant' endogenous dermatitis has to be elucidated: the term 'post-exogenous eczema' or 'persistent occupational dermatitis' is more appropriate and the

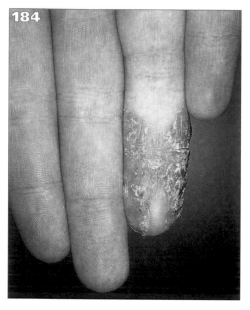

184 Post-occupational dermatitis in a cook with an atopic background.

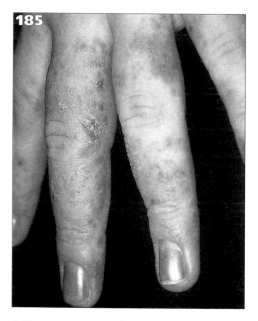

185 Dermatitis on the inner sides of the fingers in a food handler due to immediate-type reactions.

mechanism is probably comparable with that of post-traumatic eczema (184).

Key to diagnosis

Transition from capricious pattern into chronic course, continuing after cessation of exposure.

Immediate contact reaction

Itching, tingling or burning sensations with local wheal and flare reactions are the typical, and weakest, type of immediate reactions. Some compounds induce a more eczematous picture, especially in cases of chronic exposure. Most reactions occur on the inner and dorsal sides of the fingers.

At risk are employees who handle animal products, vegetables, fruits, nuts, medications or who wear latex gloves. Most immediate reactions occur in occupations where allergic and cumulative irritant dermatitis are common. Diagnosis is time consuming and difficult (185–188).

Key to diagnosis

Occupation; localisation; positive immediate-type allergy tests.

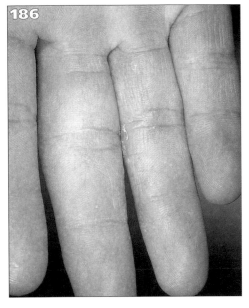

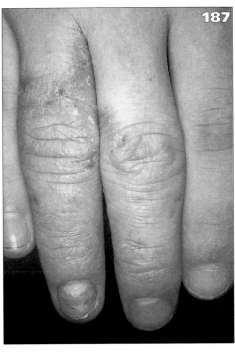

186, 187 Dermatitis on the fingers in a cook caused by immediate-type reactions to shrimps and oranges.

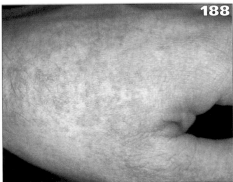

188 'Gut'-eczema in a slaughterhouse operative due to immediate-type reactions to the visceral fluids of pigs.

Pompholyx

Pompholyx is an eruption of small itching vesicles on the inner and palmar sides of the fingers and palms, sometimes around nail folds, preceded by an itching or burning sensation; there is no erythema or symmetrical localisation. Patients tend to open the vesicles with their nails or needles to obtain relief from the maddening itch. Repeated eruptions may lead to inflammation and a more eczematous picture.

Pompholyx is often mistakenly regarded as an 'endogenous' dermatitis, but it occurs in both irritant and allergic contact dermatitis and in nickel-sensitised patients. It should be regarded as a

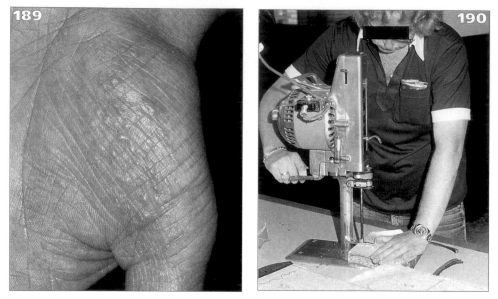

189, 190 Pompholyx-like allergic contact dermatitis due to dimethyl thiourea used as an anti-oxidant in textile patterned paper.

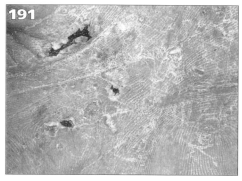

191 Pompholyx with the vesicle opened by a needle.

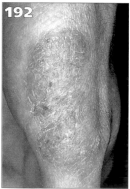

192 Discoid eczema.

physical sign rather than a diagnosis in its own right (**189–191**).

Key to diagnosis

Periodical occurrence of itching vesicles between the fingers and on the palmar sides of the hands.

Discoid eczema

Discoid, or nummular, eczema has one or more round lesions with a vesicular or scaly type of eczema; it is a chronic condition with a preference for the dorsum of the hands and fingers. It is difficult to treat, often tending to relapse. It is most common among atopics and in occupations with cumulative irritation (**192**).

Key to diagnosis

Unaffected skin between lesions and recurrence at the same location. Discoid eczema on other parts of the body.

Neurodermatitis circumscripta

This condition has a demarcated patch of lichenified eczema on the dorsum of the hands or fingers, caused by the patient rubbing the skin. It may be regarded as 'mechanical' dermatitis (193).

Key to diagnosis

Lichenification; history.

Phototoxic and photoallergic reactions

A photodermatitis may vary from burning redness to a typical eczema (see Chapter 4). Photodermatitis occurs on the light-exposed skin areas and so is determined by the type of clothes the patient wears. Most reactions occur on the face, neck, arms and hands. Photoreactions are induced by a combination of irradiation and skin contact with an exogenous compound or in combination with a systemic administered compound. Phytophototoxic dermatitis (see Chapter 7) is characterised by a sharply demarcated redness that may become bullous and typically cause hyperpigmentation.

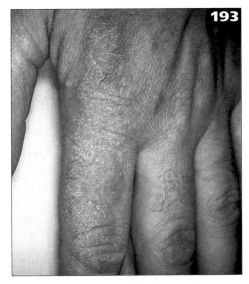

193 Neurodermatitis circumscripta.

In general, phototoxic reactions mimic sunburn, photoallergic reactions having an eczematous aspect. The patient's history is very important to detect exposure to exogenous compounds or the use of systemic or topical medications (194, 195).

Key to diagnosis

Exposure to sun; localisation; garden activities.

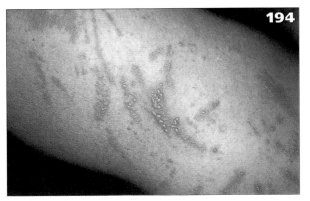

194 Phytophotodermatitis.

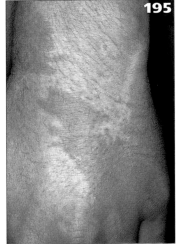

195 Allergic contact dermatitis with sharp demarcation due to industrial sensitisation to ethylenediamine.

Various dermatoses

Some common or rare dermatoses may cause eruptions that mimic hand eczema. Examples are acrodermatitis enteropath-ica, lichen planus, lupus erythematosus, warts and granuloma annulare (**196, 197**).

Key to diagnosis

Histopathology.

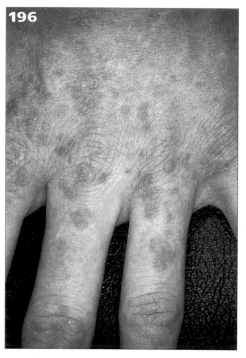

196 Plane warts.

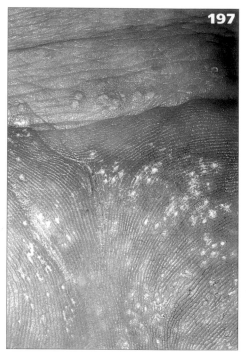

197 Lichen planus.

BIBLIOGRAPHY

Menne, T and Maibach, HI (1993), *Hand Eczema*, CRC Press, Boca Raton.
Rook, A, Wilkinson, DS and Ebling, FJG (1992), *Textbook of Dermatology*, Blackwell Scientific Publications, Oxford.
Rycroft, RJG, Menne, T and Frosch, PJ (1995), *Textbook of Contact Dermatitis*, Springer-Verlag, Berlin.

CHAPTER SEVEN

OCCUPATIONAL DERMATITIS DUE TO PLANTS AND WOODS

Christopher R Lovell

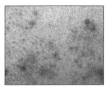

Irritant dermatitis from contact with a prickly pear; it can resemble scabies.

Daffodil picker's dermatitis.

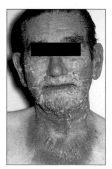

Air-borne allergic contact dermatitis from cutting down trees.

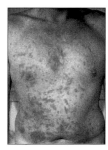

Linear lesions are pathogno-monic of contact with plants; this was phytophotoder-matitis.

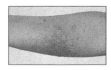

Rhus dermatitis is common in the US.

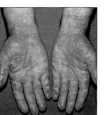

Allergy from *Compositae* should be suspected in seasonal hand eczema.

INTRODUCTION

Our lives are inextricably tangled with the plant kingdom. We depend on plants for food and there are few homes, offices or factories not graced by ornamental pot plants. In addition, many occupations are particularly at risk from exposure to hazardous plants or plant products. Some examples are listed in *Table 17*. In a Swedish series, floristry and horticulture ranked 11th for women and 13th for men in the frequency of occupational causes of dermatitis. Agriculture and forestry are also major causes of occupational skin disease throughout the world.

Plants may adversely affect the skin in a variety of ways, some an intentional part of the plant's defence mechanism to prevent it being eaten or gathered. More commonly, the adverse reaction is to a substance or structure which is produced by the plant for another purpose, e.g. to reduce susceptibility to fungal attack. A classification of adverse reactions to plants is given in *Table 18*. It should be remembered that dermatitis attributed to plants may be due to other causes, for example as a contact allergy from protective rubber gloves, allergic or irritant reactions to garden chemicals, or urticated eruptions caused by the stinging hairs of certain caterpillar species (e.g. the brown-tail moth, *Euproctis chrysorrhoea*).

Table 17. Occupations exposed to plants and woods.

Gardeners; nursery workers; fruit pickers

Florists; flower arrangers; greengrocers

Farmers; agriculturalists

Foresters; sawyers; lumberjacks

Carpenters; wood machinists; builders

Antique restorers; musical instrument makers; musicians

Botanists; naturalists

Aromatherapists; herbalists; homoeopaths

Plant biochemists; pharmacologists; pharmacists

Dentists; vets; dermatologists

Perfumiers; cosmetologists; beauticians

Food handlers; chefs; bar staff

Professional sportsmen

Military personnel on exercise

Climbers; outward bound instructors

Table 18. Adverse reactions to plants.

Irritant: mechanical and/or chemical

Urticating: pharmacological/immunological

Phototoxic

Allergic

IRRITANT REACTIONS

Irritancy caused by plants may be due to either mechanical or chemical factors or a mixture of both. In certain occupations, irritant reactions caused by plants may be compounded by other irritants such as wet work in floristry or food handling. Many plants possess rough hairs on the surface of the leaves and stems, sometimes even sharp spines. These are designed partly to reduce the chance of predation from browsing animals and also sometimes to trap water or to deflect water away from certain parts of the plant. Minor chemical irritation is common – many people will notice a slight tingling of the fingertips after pricking out their tomato plant seedlings. However, irritation may be more severe. Most people will take care to avoid the formidable spines on many cacti and succulents such as *Yucca*. However, certain cactus species, including *Opuntia*, have tiny clusters of hairs (called glochids) on their pads. *Opuntia* species include the prickly pear (**198**); individuals harvesting the fruit may develop a papular, intensely itchy eruption somewhat resembling scabies, so-called 'sabra dermatitis' (**199**).

Sometimes the selection of more vigorous cultivars of a plant may increase the risk of irritant exposure; thus the ornamental shrub *Fremontodendron* was for many years grown as a choice specimen near the sunny walls of stately homes. However, new cultivars, including 'California Glory' (**200**), are freely available from garden centres. When the plant is handled, it showers a huge quantity of brownish hairs which microscopically look like sea urchins and are intensely irritant.

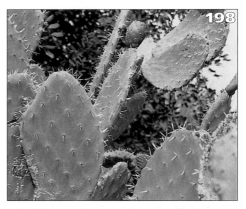

198 The prickly pear, *Opuntia ficus-indica*, grown as a boundary marker.

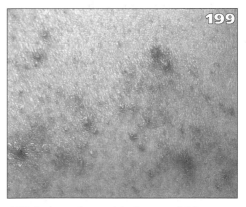

199 Irritant dermatitis due to prickly pear.

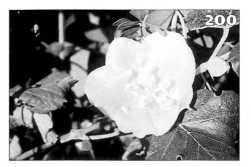

200 *Fremontodendron* cv. 'California Glory'.

105

Many irritant plant species present a relatively minor problem in individuals who cultivate small numbers but when handled in bulk the mechanical irritancy is compounded, thus mass cultivation of borage (**201**) for its essential oil may induce irritant reactions in those harvesting the plant. Mechanical procedures such as trimming chicory or milling herbs (**202**) will also enhance the irritant effect.

The sap of many plant species is intensely irritant due to a variety of chemicals including calcium oxalate, present in many bulb species such as *Allium* (onions and garlic), *Tulipia* (tulips) and *Narcissus* (daffodils) (**203**); nurserymen and florists who handle daffodil bulbs or cut stems typically present with fingertip dermatitis (**204**). Individuals handling vegetables such as chicory (**205**) may develop a similar skin reaction. Chicory is also an allergen.

Several irritant species are found in the genus *Euphorbia* (spurge), named after Euphorbus, a Numidian physician. These include some garden weeds such as the petty spurge but also ornamental species such as *Euphorbia marginata* (**206**) which is popular among flower arrangers, particularly in Japan. The sap from *Euphorbia* species contains, among other substances, irritant phorbol esters. Minor trauma to the plant will release this irritant sap as shown in **207**. Several species of *Euphorbia*,

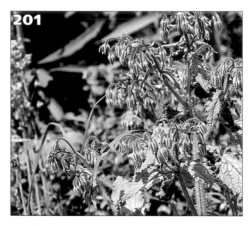

201 Borage (*Borago officinalis*).

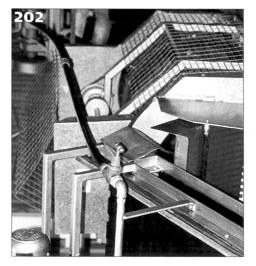

202 Milling parsley.

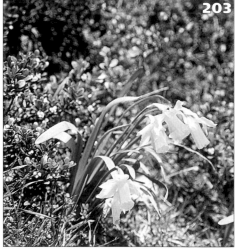

203 *Narcissus pseudonarcissus*.

including *Euphorbia myrsinites*, are grown as ornamental garden plants and gardeners may develop severe irritant contact dermatitis, causing eyelid oedema which mimics allergic dermatitis (**208**); sap in the eyes may even cause blindness. Most succulent *Euphorbia* species are relatively innocuous, however, attempts to cultivate one species, *E. tirucalli*, as a 'green' source of hydrocarbon fuel were abandoned because of the severe irritancy in operatives.

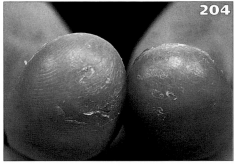

204 Fingertip dermatitis in a daffodil handler.

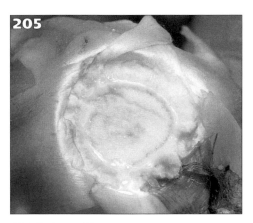

205 Irritant chicory sap.

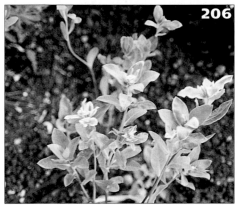

206 *Euphorbia marginata* ('Snow in summer'), commonly used in floristry.

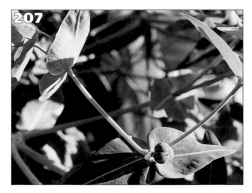

207 Traumatised *Euphorbia* showing white sap leaking from the broken stem.

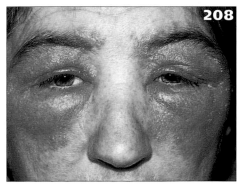

208 Severe irritant dermatitis due to *Euphorbia myrsinites* in a gardener.

Dieffenbachia picta (the dumb cane) is a commonly grown office plant which can also cause severe irritant dermatitis and even blindness. Bundles of needle-like crystals (raphides) held within plant cells are ejected forcibly after contact with water. *Dieffenbachia* can be fatal if ingested.

Correct identification of the plants handled should enable a diagnosis of irritant contact dermatitis and, if the plant is a known irritant, it should not be used in patch testing routinely as patch tests may induce chemical burns and even keloid scars. Mild mechanical irritation is often self-limiting. Careful hand washing and the use of protective gloves when handling plant material will usually prevent significant chemical irritation, and, as with other forms of dermatitis, barrier creams are of dubious value. If hairs or spines are implanted in the skin, they can often be removed by Sellotape stripping.

URTICARIA

Urticaria caused by plants is sometimes due to urticant chemicals inoculated by the plant. A typical example is the stinging nettle, *Urtica dioica*, although several other species similarly induce urticaria and some of these, such as *Loasa* and *Caiophora*, are being increasingly grown as ornamentals by specialist nurserymen. Occupational urticaria is more commonly and importantly due to immediate hypersensitivity to a substance, usually a protein, on the surface of the plant. This condition often, but not exclusively, affects atopics. Currently, probably the most significant botanical cause of urticaria is the rubber tree, *Hevea brasiliensis* – surface proteins on latex products can cause severe urticaria, anaphylaxis and even death in individuals who handle them, including medical and nursing personnel.

Other plant products inducing urticaria include henna, a plant derived dye, a cause of urticaria and even anaphylaxis in hairdressers. Food handlers are at particular risk of urticaria and 'protein contact dermatitis' due to type 1 allergy from vegetable products. Some of the important causes are listed in *Table 19*. Important species include mustard, *Brassica oleracea* (**209**), paprika, lettuce and strawberries.

Sometimes an individual can react to one part of the plant and not to another, for example, potato peel but not the flesh of the potato tuber. Careful prick testing to fresh vegetables handled at work can be rewarding (**210**) but it is essential that adequate resuscitation facilities are available, although the risk is very slight with this procedure.

Table 19. Immunological urticaria due to plants and plant products.

Food handlers: various beans; vegetables (e.g. lettuce); fruit; spices (e.g. mustard; paprika)
Perfumiers/beauticians: lime extract; balsams of Peru; sesame seed oil
Hairdressers: henna
Cotton growers
Health professionals: latex
Hardwood handlers: teak, etc.
Gardeners; plantsmen: tulips; iris, etc.

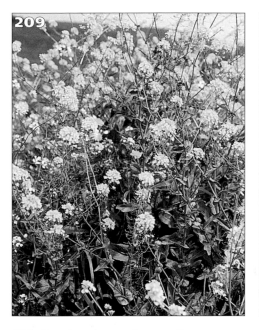

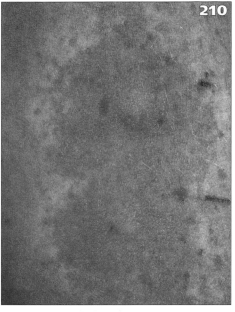

209 *Brassica oleracea* (mustard).

210 Positive prick tests to fresh vegetables.

PHOTOTOXIC REACTIONS

Phototoxic reactions are caused by plants belonging to a relatively small number of families (*Table 20*). The phototoxic substances – psoralens – are natural fungicides in the plant, thus a plant which is showing early signs of decay may release higher amounts of psoralens. Paradoxically, a very healthy, organically grown plant may contain more psoralens than a plant grown by standard techniques. The production of new, disease-free cultivars of plants may result in increased concentrations of psoralens, putting horticulturists at risk. Finally, the production of new strains of vegetables such as parsnips, which can now be harvested during the sunnier months of the year, will be more likely to produce phototoxic reactions in individuals handling them.

Table 20. Plant families causing phototoxic reactions.

Umbelliferae
Vegetables, e.g. celery; carrot; fennel; parsnip
Herbs, e.g. dill; angelica; chervil; cumin; parsley; lovage
Ornamentals, e.g. Queen Anne's lace (*Ammi majus*)
Weeds, e.g. cow parsnip; hogweed

Rutaceae
Citrus fruit, e.g. bergamot; orange; lemon
Rue
Dictamnus (burning bush)

Moraceae
Fig

Leguminosae
Psoralea corylifolia (bavchi)

The constituent psoralens react with the DNA of mammalian cells forming cross-links. Irradiation with long-wave ultraviolet light (UVA) produces thymine dimers which disrupt and prevent normal replication of the DNA. In the skin the eruption is typically linear (due to brushing against the plant) bullous and often exquisitely tender. Classically, the lesions are followed by hyperpigmentation as the blisters resolve (**211**, **212**). Rarely, hypopigmentation may follow.

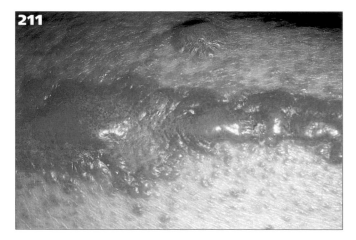

211 Bullous phototoxic reaction.

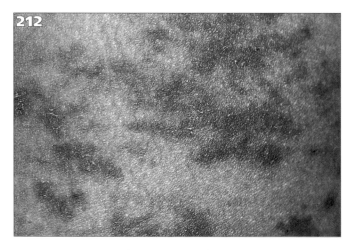

212 Hyperpigmented areas in a resolving phytophototoxic reaction.

The most common ornamental plant to cause this reaction is rue (*Ruta graveolens*) (**213**) and in the United States *Dictamnus albus* (**214**), the burning bush. In sunny autumns, fig pickers may develop phototoxic reactions from the broken parts of the plant *Ficus carica* (**215**). Similarly, individuals who harvest citrus fruit, such as oranges and limes, are at risk.

Numerous occupations are at risk of phototoxic reactions some of which are listed in *Table 21*.

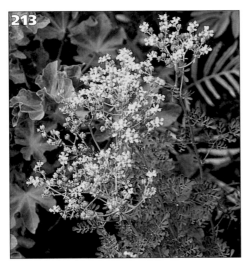

213 Garden rue (*Ruta graveolens*).

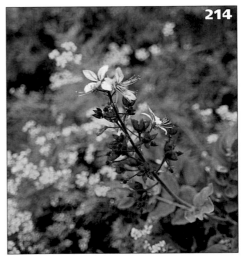

214 *Dictamnus albus*, the gas plant or burning bush, growing at the Oxford Botanic Garden.

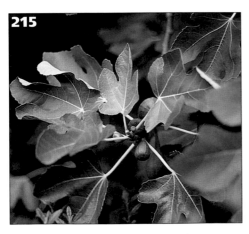

215 Fig, *Ficus carica*; immature fruit.

Table 21. Occupations and activities at risk of phototoxic reactions.

Gardening:
rue; *Dictamnus*; parsnip
use of string trimmers
harvesting figs and citrus fruit

Canning or processing vegetables

Fishermen

Sportsmen (e.g. swimmers)

Military on exercise

111

Many vegetables, including parsnips, parsley and celery, are rich in psoralens, hence individuals who process celery for canning when it is past its best (**216**) are particularly at risk of phototoxicity. Certain gardening tools, such as string trimmers, deliver a buckshot spray of plant sap at the operator (**217, 218**); several plants attacked in this way include members of the *Umbelliferae*, such as cow parsnip and cow parsley (**219**). If the operator is scantily clad, the phototoxic reaction presents as a series of erythematous and then hyperpigmented macules which may mimic other cutaneous disorders such as pityriasis lichenoides (**220**). However, the operator's back and covered sites are spared, unlike in the latter condition.

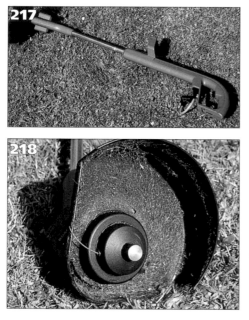

216 Decaying celery.

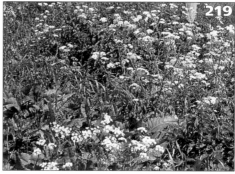

219 Cow parsley (*Anthriscus sylvestris*) growing wild.

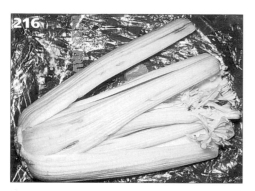

217, 218 String trimmer.

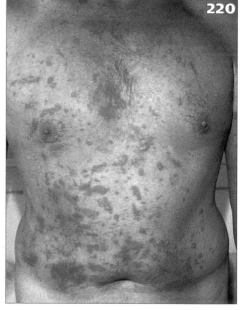

220 String trimmer dermatitis, also described as 'strimmer rash' and 'weed wackers' dermatitis'.

PREVENTIVE MEASURES

Phototoxic reactions should be entirely preventable. Species such as rue should not be planted near swimming pools or other areas where contact with bare skin is likely. Individuals operating strimmers should be clothed or work in the evenings or cloudy weather. UVA protectant sunscreens have been shown to reduce phototoxic reactions in parsley pickers.

ALLERGIC DERMATITIS

Several plant species have been reported as causing allergic contact dermatitis, however, many such case reports are solitary and only a relatively small proportion of plants present a major problem. It appears that allergic dermatitis is more common than irritant dermatitis in florists and gardeners; delayed hypersensitivity depends on the individual's susceptibility to certain molecules. The most important allergenic molecular groups are listed in *Table 22*.

In the United States, particularly on the Eastern seaboard, poison ivy (*Rhus*) dermatitis is a major cause of severe allergic reactions in horticulturists, gardeners, farmers and foresters. Several species of *Rhus* (*Toxicodendron*) are allergenic. They include the poison ivy, Rhus radicans (**221**), which causes a florid bullous eruption (**222**); severe reactions may

Table 22. Major plant allergens.

Urushiols (poison ivy; *Grevillea*)
Sesquiterpene lactones (daisy family)
Quinones (primula; *Streptocarpus*; orchids; hardwoods)
Falcarinols (ivy; carrot)
Usnic acid (lichens)
Abietic acid derivatives (colophony)

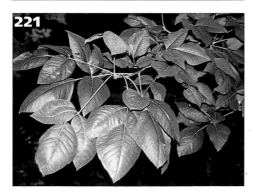

221 Poison ivy (*Rhus radicans*).

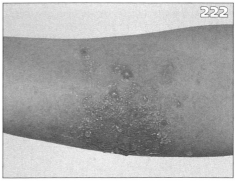

222 Bullous allergic contact dermatitis from *Rhus* species in a North American nursery worker.

113

result in systemic illness, secondary infection and even death. The allergens are present in the sticky sap of the plant so rapid washing of the skin after contact can help reduce the severity of the reaction. Attempts at desensitisation have not proven helpful to date. Other members of the family Anacardiaceae are also potent sensitisers – occupations at risk include mango pickers, oriental lacquer craftsmen and cashew nut processors.

A major cause of allergic contact dermatitis in florists is the genus *Alstroemeria*, the so-called Peruvian Lily (223). This is an ideal cut plant as it is extremely long lasting. However, the stems are leafy and the leaves need to be stripped away from the plant. Individual flowers are also used in wreaths and corsages, resulting in maximum exposure to the florist's skin. Typically, *Alstroemeria* dermatitis affects the fingertips (224, 225) although other sites, such as eyelids,

may also be involved. The same allergen, called tuliposide A, is found in tulips. Allergic dermatitis, 'tulip fingers', is common in The Netherlands and Scandinavia, affecting bulb growers, diggers, sorters and packers as well as the actual flower pickers. Finger stalls (cots) may be helpful.

The mass production of florists' chrysanthemums (*X. Dendranthema*) (226) is an important cause of dermatitis, particularly in The Netherlands and Denmark. In order to obtain bushy plants, the main bud is broken off ('disbudding'); this encourages the growth of lateral shoots (227). This procedure has to be done manually and is a major cause of fingertip dermatitis. The dermatitis may also extent to the forearm (228) and face, chiefly via fingertip contamination, although volatile allergens and volatile material from the surface of the plant may also contribute to facial dermatitis.

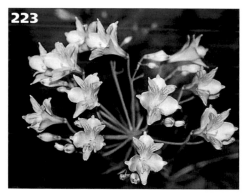

223 Peruvian Lily.

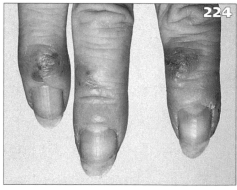

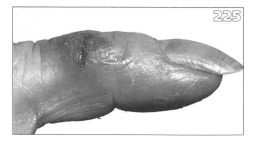

224, 225 Fingertip dermatitis due to *Alstroemeria* in a florist.

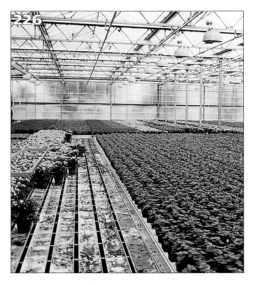

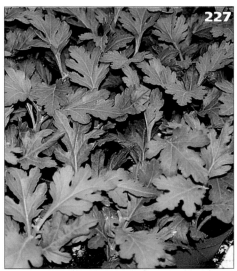

226 Mass production of florists' chrysanthemums in Denmark.

227 'Disbudded' chrysanthemums.

228 Allergic dermatitis from chrysanthemums (usually seasonal).

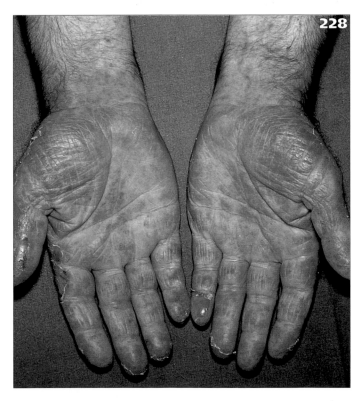

Other members of the daisy family (Compositae) are also allergenic. **229** shows an example of facial dermatitis caused by dandelion in a gardener. Operating lawn mowers or power tools releases sap from the injured plants, spraying the operator. Unlike photosensitivity, allergic contact dermatitis can involve the palms and finger webs (**230**) together with relatively sun-protected sites such as nasolabial folds and behind the ears. However, individuals with chronic allergic contact dermatitis due to members of the daisy family may also subsequently develop photosensitive dermatitis ('chronic actinic dermatitis'). Chemically similar allergens are found in liverworts, such as *Frullania*, a major cause of 'airborne' pattern allergic dermatitis in forestry workers in several parts of the world, notably continental Europe and Canada. Several lichens induce a similar pattern in harvesters.

Primula obconica (**231**) is one of the most common domestic causes of allergic contact dermatitis. Generally, florists and gardeners are aware of the hazards from the plant and so it is a rarer occupational cause. However, **232** shows cheilitis in a nursery worker who is allergic to *Primula obconica* and who licked her fingers after pricking out seedlings.

Colophony, the major allergen in sticking plaster, is derived from species of pine and other conifers and may elicit allergic contact dermatitis in colophony-

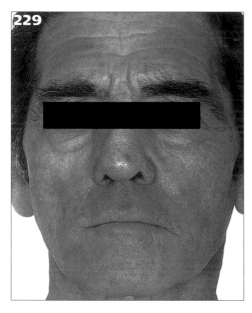

229 Facial dandelion dermatitis.

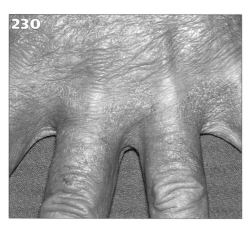

230 Compositae dermatitis involving sites shielded from sun exposure.

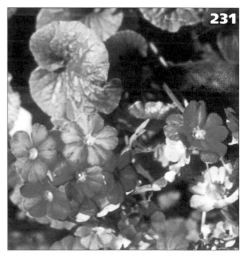

231 *Primula obconica.*

sensitive individuals. The major culprit is the rapidly growing Leyland cypress (*X.Cupressocyparis leylandii*) which can cause severe airborne facial dermatitis in gardeners who chop down or burn the plant material (**233**). Sprigs used in floristry may also induce allergic contact dermatitis.

232 Allergic cheilitis in a nursery worker who handled *Primula obconica.*

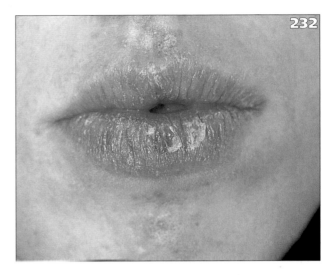

233 Facial dermatitis in a gardener who cut down and burnt *X Cupressocyparis leylandii.*

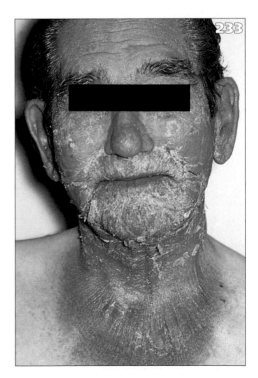

Several hardwood trees are allergenic but many of the species are now extremely vulnerable in the wild and so are less commonly used in the furniture industry. However, a few specialist antique restorers still handle small amounts of tropical hardwoods and even these small amounts may sensitise. Recorder makers may be sensitised to rosewoods and blackwood. A few other hardwoods, including iroko, are still quite commonly used for window frames, etc., putting carpenters and joiners at particular risk. Some of the more commonly encountered allergenic hardwoods are listed in *Table 23*.

Patch testing to sawdust from hardwoods will often elicit irritant reactions and may sensitise a patient, and should only be carried out with care in specialist departments. A positive patch test reaction is shown in **234**. Wood dust may cause an airborne contact dermatitis **235**. **236** shows a dermatitis on the forearms after the individual rested his arms on an iroko window frame.

Table 23. The more common allergenic hardwoods.

Eucalyptus spp. (gum)
Olea europaea (olive)
Khaya spp. (African mahogany)
Gluta/Melanorrhoea spp. (Rengas wood)
Acacia melanoxylon (Australian black wood)
Dalbergia spp. (some rosewoods; African blackwood)
Machaerium scleroxylon (Pao ferro)
Tectonia grandis (teak)
Chlorophora excelsa (iroko)

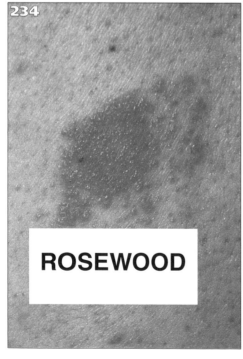

234 Positive patch test in a wood handler.

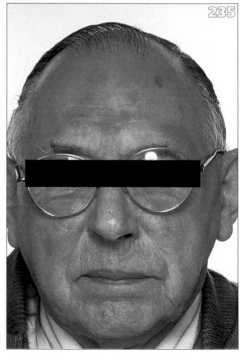

235 Airborne contact dermatitis from wood dust.

PREVENTIVE MEASURES

The management of hardwood dermatitis includes primary prevention. For example, the workforce should be warned of potentially hazardous woods (unfortunately much timber is imported inaccurately or imprecisely labelled) and work areas should be adequately ventilated. 'Damping down' dust will reduce allergenicity as well as the fire hazard.

A precise diagnosis of allergic contact dermatitis can only be made by careful patch testing so it is essential that individuals are not tested by a huge variety of plant parts as there is a high risk of sensitisation. Fortunately, an increasing number of allergens are commercially available; this reduces the risk of sensitisation, can give more standardised results and enable exclusion of the commoner plant allergens. The list, however, is far from complete and it may be necessary to patch test with the plant itself. Before doing this, however, it is essential to ensure that the plant is not a major irritant or does not cause severe toxic reactions by cutaneous absorption; correct and precise identification of the plant is always essential.

Often, precise identification of the allergen can be curative, enabling the individual to avoid a known plant species. In occupations such as floristry, where it is difficult to avoid genera such as Alstroemeria, heavy-duty nitrile gloves may help to reduce the degree of exposure.

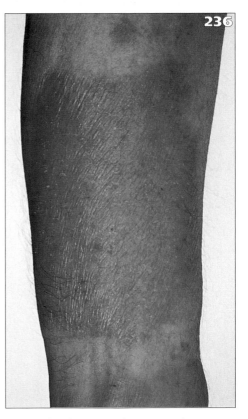

236 Iroko dermatitis from a window frame.

BIBLIOGRAPHY

Rycroft, RJG (1993), Occupational exposure to plants, *Plants and the Skin*, Blackwell Scientific Publications, Oxford, 6–15.

CHAPTER EIGHT

OCCUPATIONAL ACNE

Craig Omohundro and James S Taylor

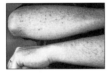

Oil folliculitis.

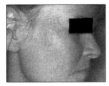

Chloracne in a spouse in contact with the worker's overalls.

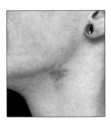

Localised occlusive acne due to a violon chin rest.

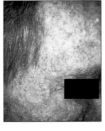

Severe chloracne.

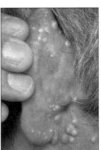

Straw-coloured cysts behind the ear are pathognomonic of chloracne.

2,3,7,8-Tetrachlorodibenzo-p-dioxin (TCDD) is notorious for causing chloracne.

INTRODUCTION

Occupational acne is a variety of acne venenata resulting from various chemical exposures as well as from a variety of environmental physical and mechanical factors encountered in the workplace. The eruption may be mild, involving localised exposure or covered areas of the body, or severe, explosive and disseminated with the involvement of almost every follicular orifice (**237, 238**). Additionally, chloracne almost always represents a cutaneous sign of systemic exposure to highly toxic chemicals. In general, occupational acne is separated into oil acne, chloracne, coal tar acne, acne cosmetica, acne aestivalis, acne mechanica, and tropical acne. This listing is not intended to be exhaustive but may serve as a useful paradigm and includes the most common causes of occupational acne.

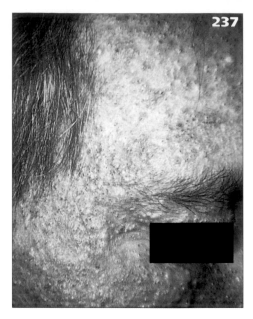

237 Severe chloracne from chlorbenzenes involving almost every follicular orifice of the face.

OIL ACNE

Oil acne is the most common form of occupational acne and is most frequently observed in individuals employed in the machine tooling trades. Its incidence has decreased in recent years, however, probably due to the automation of tooling machines and to improved industrial hygiene conditions in the workplace.

Cutting oils, especially the neat oils, and semisynthetic metalworking fluids have been the most commonly incriminated oil acnegens. In addition, prolonged exposure to grease and lubricating oils, as occurs in auto, truck and aircraft mechanics, may induce oil acne; kerosene has also been reported to be acnegenic. Other workers potentially affected with oil acne include oil well drillers, textile mill workers, petroleum refiners and rubber workers.

Acne which has been observed in young fast-food workers exposed to grease and fat while frying hamburgers has been dubbed 'McDonald's acne' although there is little evidence that this is a separate entity.

Prolonged oil exposure produces a reactive follicular hyperkeratosis and results in sebum retention. This manifests clinically as multiple open comedones, inflammatory folliculitis and microcystic lesions caused by the oil itself, primarily distributed over exposed areas such as the dorsal hands and extensor forearms (**239**). Oil-soaked clothing may produce lesions on the thighs, lower abdomen and buttocks, as well as the face from wiping the brow with an oil contaminated sleeve (**240**). Inflammatory lesions ('oil boils')

238 Severe chloracne on the buttocks in a laboratory research scientist.

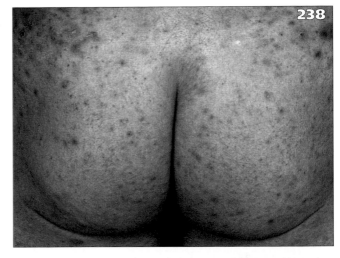

239 Oil folliculitis with follicular plugging and inflammatory papules (courtesy of the National Institute for Occupational Safety and Health, Cincinnati, OH).

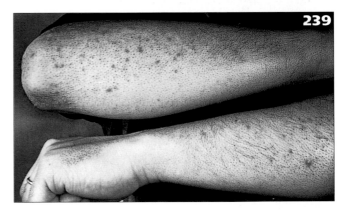

240 Localised acne on the face of an apprentice engineer from wiping the brow with an oil soaked sleeve.

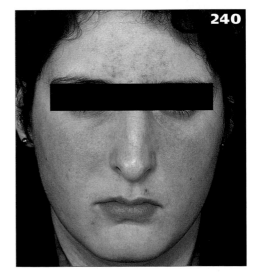

are more prominent than in chloracne and may mimic conglobate cystic acne.

Oil acne is not caused by bacteria growing in metalworking fluids. It is treated with the usual acne vulgaris modalities such as topical benzoyl peroxide and retinoic acid. Systemic treatment is often needed with tetracycline, erythromycin or minocycline, or with isotretinoin in severe cases. The key factor is avoiding contact with oils and grease. Work clothes should be changed daily and frequent cleansing of the skin with soap and water is advised.

CHLORACNE (HALOGEN ACNE)

Chloracne results from environmental exposure to certain halogenated aromatic hydrocarbons and is considered to be one of the most sensitive indicators of systemic poisoning by these compounds.

Chloracne was first observed by von Bettman in 1897 and by Herxheimer in 1899. Since then a number of chloracnegenic chemicals have been identified. Prior to World War II, most cases were thought to be caused by chloronaphthalenes and polychlorinated biphenyls (PCBs). More recently, trace contaminants formed during the manufacture of PCBs and other polychlorinated compounds, especially herbicides, have been causally linked to chloracne development. These include polyhalogenated dibenzofurans in association with PCBs, polychlorinated dibenzo-*p*-dioxins and chlorinated azo- and azoxybenzenes which are contaminants of 3,4-dichloraniline and related herbicides.

Interestingly, chloracnegenic compounds are structurally similar, all sharing relative molecular planarity and containing two benzene rings with halogen atoms occupying at least three of the lateral ring positions. The position of halogen substitution appears to be critical, as substitution at positions that lead to molecular non-planarity reduces biological activity. Stereo-specific binding of these compounds to a receptor is implicated in their toxicity.

Most cases of chloracne have resulted from occupational exposure in chemical manufacturing or rarely from end-use of products. Exposure is usually through direct contact but inhalation and ingestion may also be operative in some cases.

Non-occupational chloracne has resulted from industrial accidents, contaminated industrial waste, and contaminated food products. A widely publicised example was the extensive environmental contamination with the compound 2,3,7,8-tetrachlorodibenzo-*p*-dioxin (TCDD) (**241**) which occurred on 10 July 1976 at the ICMESA chemical plant near Seveso, Italy. During production of trichlorophenol, an explosion resulted in the formation and ultimate discharge into the atmosphere of an estimated two kilograms of TCDD. The contaminated area encompassed more than 200 acres (81 ha) of land; 135 cases of chloracne, mostly in children, were confirmed among some 2000 inhabitants.

Other examples are the widespread ingestion of tainted rice cooking oil that occurred in Japan in 1968 and in Taiwan in 1979. Popular brands of oil were contaminated with PCBs and dibenzofurans resulting in the largest epidemics of chloracne to date. Over 1000 patients were affected with 'oil disease' called Yusho in Japan, and Yucheng in Taiwan.

For a list of known chloracnegens see *Table 24*. Of related interest, *Table 25*

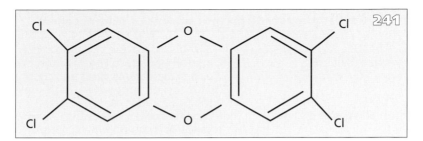

241 2,3,7,8-Tetrachlorodibenzo-*p*-dioxin (TCDD) – a halogenated aromatic compound – is highly toxic and causes chloracne.

Table 24. Chloracne-producing chemicals (chloracnegens).

Polyhalogenated naphthalenes:[1]

polychloronaphthalenes
polybromonaphthalenes[2,3]

Polyhalogenated biphenyls:

polychlorobiphenyls (PCBs)
polybromodiphenyls (PBBs)

Polyhalogenated dibenzofurans:[1]

polychlorodibenzofurans, especially tri-, tetra-, penta- and hexachlorodibenzofuran
polybromodibenzofurans, especially tetrabromodibenzofuran

Contaminants of polychlorophenol compounds, especially herbicides (2,4,5-T and pentachlorophenol) and herbicide intermediates (2,4,5-trichlorophenol):

2,3,7,8-tetrachlorodibenzo-*p*-dioxin (TCDD)
hexachlorodibenzo-*p*-dioxin
tetrachlorodibenzofuran

Contaminants of 3,4-dichloroaniline and related herbicides:

3,4,3',4'-tetrachloroazoxybenzene (TCAOB)
3,4,3',4'-tetrachloroazobenzene (TCAB)

Other:

1,2,3,4-tetrachlorobenzene (experimental)
Dichlobenil, a herbicide (clinical only)
DDT (crude trichlorobenzene[3])

1 The polychlorodibenzofurans and hexachloronaphthalenes may occur as contaminants in some PCBs.
2 The polybromonaphthalenes may occur as contaminants in some PBBs.
3 Not confirmed as chloracnegens.

Table 25. Partial list of past and present sources of chloracnegens.

Chloracnegen	Source
Polychloronaphthalenes	Electrical insulators; fire-resistant materials; wood preservatives; boat hull coatings (antimagnetic properties); high-pressure additives for lubricants
Polychlorobiphenyls (PCBs)	Hydraulic fluids; plastics; adhesives; fire retardants in transformers; sealants
Polychlorodibenzofurans (PCDFs)	Contaminants of PCBs and various chlorinated phenols
Polychlorinated phenols	Wood preservatives; leather; paper industry applications; herbicides; fungicides; algicides; insecticides; disinfectants
Dioxins	Contaminant of Agent Orange, formed during production of chlorinated organic solvents (hexachlorophene and the herbicide 2,4,5,-T); products of combustion
Azo- and azoxybenzenes	Herbicide intermediates

provides a partial list of past and present sources of the various chloracnegens.

Clinically, chloracne is characterised by multiple closed comedones and straw-coloured cysts distributed over the malar crescents (**242–245**) and retroauricular folds (**246, 247**), typically with sparing of the nose. Inflammatory lesions occur but are less frequent than in other forms of acne. As toxicity increases, the posterior neck, trunk and extremities (**248–250**), buttocks, scrotum, and penis (**238, 251**) may become involved.

Cutaneous findings occasionally associated with chloracne, which may point to certain exposures, include hyperpigmentation of the skin (PCBs; TCDD), hyperpigmentation of the nails (**252**) and mucous membranes (PCBs), follicular hyperkeratosis (PCBs; TCDD, as at Seveso), conjunctivitis and meibomian gland changes (PCBs), facial erythema and oedema (trichlorophenol), hypertrichosis (TCDD), hyperhidrosis of the palms and soles (TCDD; PCBs), folliculitis and xerosis (TCAB; TCAOB) and actinic elastosis (TCDD). The erythema associated with trichlorophenol production was also seen in the Seveso cases with erythema and oedema of exposed areas (face and limbs). These 'prechloracne' lesions were also accompanied by vesiculobullous and necrotic lesions on the palms and fingertips, and papulonodular lesions, all of which disappeared within a few weeks. Hyperkeratotic, infiltrative erythematous granuloma annulare or erythema elevatum diutinum-like lesions were also seen in Seveso in association with the chloracne appearing later (two months after the explosion).

Axillary involvement and follicular hyperkeratosis are thought to be associated with the inhalation or ingestion of chloracnegens. Chloracne may occur in relatives of workers exposed at home to contaminated clothes and tools (**253**).

Histopathologically, lesions usually show squamous metaplasia and plugging of infundibular ducts as well as atrophy of sebaceous glands. However, the specificity of these findings is unclear. The rapid transformation of sebaceous glands into comedones is characteristic of chloracne. Additionally, in Seveso, eccrine duct metaplasia with possible acrosyringeal

242 Comedonal chloracne involving the malar crescent (courtesy of D.J. Gawkrodger, Sheffield, UK).

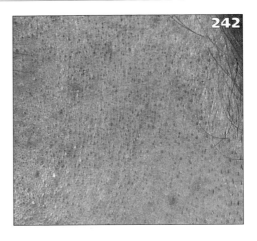

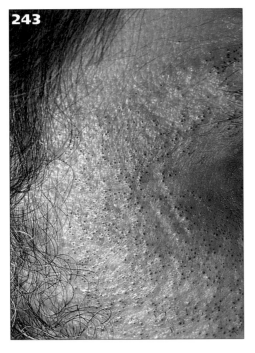

243 Comedonal chloracne of the malar crescent from chlorobenzene exposure.

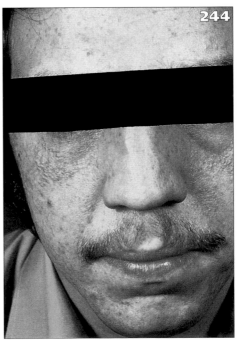

244 Chloracne of the face with straw-coloured cysts, comedones and papules (courtesy of D.J. Gawkrodger, Sheffield, UK).

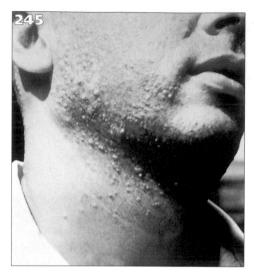

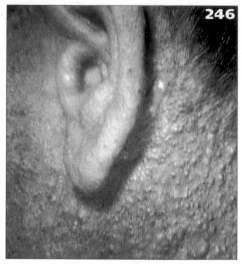

245 Chloracne with straw-coloured cysts during trichlorophenol manufacture (courtesy of National Institute for Occupational Safety and Health, Cincinnati, OH).

246 Severe retroauricular chloracne (same patient as in 237).

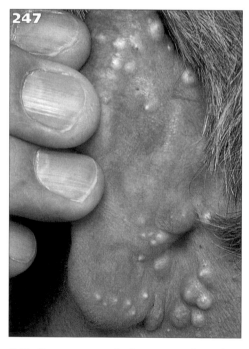

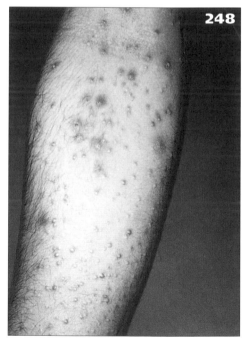

247 Gross retroauricular straw-coloured cysts (same patient as in 238).

248 Chlorobenzene chloracne of the arm with cysts and inflammatory papules.

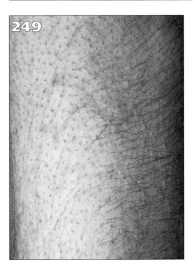

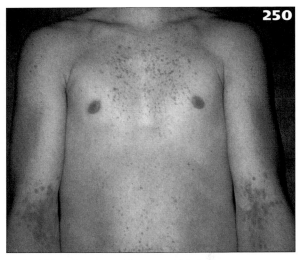

249 Chlorobenzene chloracne of the arm with follicular plugging.

250 Chlorobenzene chloracne with inflammatory papules and cysts involving the chest, abdomen and antecubital fossa.

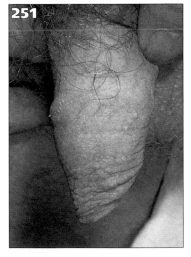

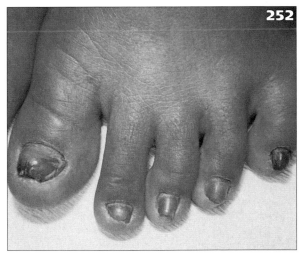

251 Chlorobenzene chloracne with papules and inflammatory cysts of the penis.

252 Hyperpigmentation, onychauxis and increased curvature of the third toenail in a six-year-old child exposed transplacentally to PCBs in Taiwan.

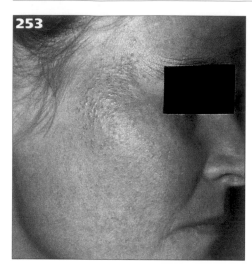

253 Chlorobenzene chloracne in the wife of a factory worker as a result of washing contaminated clothes at home.

Table 26. Clinical features of acne vulgaris vs chloracne (after Peter Pochi).

Clinical features	Acne vulgaris	Chloracne
Usual age	Teenage	Any
Comedones	Present	>3 (if absent, not chloracne)
Straw-coloured cysts	Rare	Pathognomonic
Temporal comedones	Rare	Diagnostic
Inflammatory papules and cysts	>3	Present
Retroauricular involvement	Uncommon	Common
Nose involvement	Often spared	Often spared
Associated systemic findings	Rare	Common

Table 27. Differential diagnosis of various forms of occupational acne.

Acne	Aetiology	Location	Lesion
Chloracne	Halogenated aromatics	Malar; retroauricular; mandibular	Comedones; straw-coloured cysts (0.1–1.0 cm)
Oil folliculitis	Oil	Arms; thighs; buttocks	Erythematous; papules; pustules
Pitch acne	Tar/pitch	Exposed facial areas, especially malar	Open comedones
Tropical acne	Heat/humidity	Back; neck; buttocks; proximal extremities	Nodules, cysts

cyst formation and foreign body granulomas around detached walls of eccrine gland excretory ducts was seen.

Making the diagnosis of chloracne requires a compatible clinical picture with distribution of comedones and non-inflammatory cysts outside the typical locations of acne vulgaris, documented significant exposure to known chloracnegens and absence of other external causes. Based on cutaneous findings alone, it may be very difficult to differentiate chloracne from early acne vulgaris (*Table 26*) and senile (solar) comedones of the Favre–Racouchot syndrome. Dowling–Degos disease may also be in the clinical differential diagnosis.

Differentiation of chloracne from other types of environmental acne is listed in *Table 27*.

Although chloracne tends to slowly resolve upon cessation of exposure to chloracnegenic compounds, its duration correlates with the severity of the disease which is usually a reflection of the degree and extent of exposure. Thus, in severely exposed victims of the Yusho incident in 1968, lesions characteristic of chloracne continued to develop for as long as 14 years after the initial exposure.

Treatment has, in general, been disappointing, but the retinoids seem to hold some promise. There are anecdotal reports of the unsuccessful use of oral 13-*cis*-retinoic acid, however the early institution of retinoid therapy may prevent cyst formation. Local therapy with retinoic acid, acne surgery or dermabrasion has been reported. Light cautery following topical anaesthesia with EMLA cream has recently been used.

The prevention and control of chloracne requires a totally enclosed manufacturing process with no opportunity for direct skin contact or inhalation of the toxic chemicals – a difficult environmental engineering task. The only other alternative is to attempt to alter the chemical synthetic process to eliminate or minimise exposure to the contaminant chloracnegens.

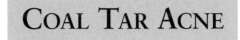

COAL TAR ACNE

Coal tar oils, creosote and pitch (especially pitch fumes) can produce a comedonal type of acne which shows a predilection for exposed areas particularly the malar regions. Cysts are infrequent, papules and pustules on covered areas may occur and lesions clear more rapidly than in chloracne. Coal tar plant workers, roofers, road maintenance workers and construction workers are among those at risk. Coal tar acne may be complicated by phototoxic reactions affecting both the skin and eyes, resulting in hyperpigmentation known as coal tar melanosis. Late complications include the development of pitch and tar papillomas (**254**), keratoses and acanthomas.

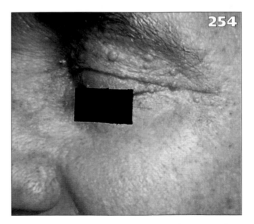

254 Hyperpigmentation, comedones and papillomas in a coal tar worker (photograph courtesy of Donald J. Birmingham).

ACNE COSMETICA

Acne cosmetica may develop in actors, actresses, and models, all of whom are often required to wear heavy, greasy make-up; cosmetologists may also be affected. This type of acne consists of essentially non-inflammatory, small, closed comedones and a few intermittent papules and pustules. When superimposed upon acne vulgaris the clinical picture may be obscured.

Many of the commonly used components of cosmetic products have been found experimentally to be comedogenic. These include lanolin, petrolatum, certain vegetable oils and pure chemicals such as butyl stearate, lauryl alcohol and oleic acid. The widespread use of such compounds may explain the high frequency of non-occupational acne cosmetica which has been estimated to affect up to one woman in three.

ACNE AESTIVALIS (MALLORCA ACNE)

Acne aestivalis is a rare, infrequently described, generally non-occupational eruption which can also affect performing artists. Typically it affects women in the age range 25–40 years and involves the cheeks, sides of the neck, chest, shoulders and upper arms. Typical lesions are erythematous, round, hard, small papules; comedones and pustules are absent or scarce. Lesions involute in the fall without scar formation. Acne aestivalis responds to topical retinoic acid but not to antibiotics.

ACNE MECHANICA

Repeated or prolonged physical insults to the skin such as rubbing, pressure, friction, pinching or pulling may produce an acneiform eruption that can be strikingly inflammatory in nature. An example is the local pressure and rubbing against seat covers that occurs in truck drivers. Other occupational causes of acne mechanica include the use of face-masks (as in hospital workers or clean-room workers in the semiconductor industry), belts, straps, tight-fitting work clothing, football shoulder pads, football helmets, hats and telephones. For acne mechanica in a violinist see **255** and **256**.

Clinically, crops of inflammatory papules and pustules appear in affected areas of skin. Deep, inflammatory nodules may result from prolonged pressure. It has been emphasised that acne mechanica is a complication of acne vulgaris and that external physical forces merely exacerbate the underlying disease locally. We have also seen it as a complication of friction and sweating in chloracne (**250**).

255, 256 Fiddler's neck: a localised acne due to the mechanical and occlusive effect of the chin rest on a violin.

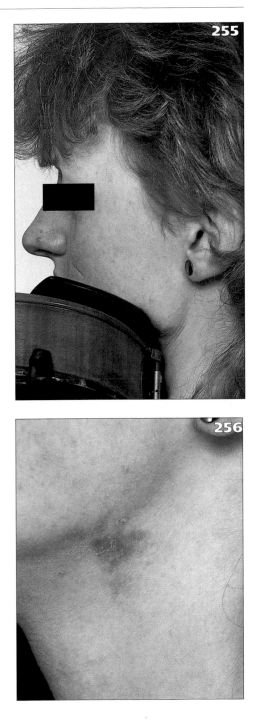

TROPICAL ACNE

BIBLIOGRAPHY

Tropical acne may result from exposure to excessively hot or humid environments; when such exposure is required for the performance of the patient's job, it may be considered as a form of occupational acne. Tropical acne has been observed most commonly in soldiers stationed in tropical climates but variants may result from chronic exposure to other hot and/or humid environments such as in foundries.

Its onset is explosive and typically occurs several months after entering the hot, humid environment. This is a severely inflammatory condition, with the development of papules, pustules, nodules and draining sinuses as in acne conglobata. Patients often feel quite ill and acute phase reactants may be elevated. There is a characteristic involvement of the buttocks and upper thighs but lesions may be extensive, with the neck, arms and trunk being affected. The face is usually spared.

Cultures have not identified a consistent pathogen, and the role of bacterial infection is felt to be unimportant. Antibiotic therapy is without significant benefit. The only effective therapeutic measure is to remove the patient from the precipitating environment.

Crow, KD (1970), Chloracne: a critical review including comparison of two series of acne from chloronaphthalene and pitch fumes, *Trans. St John's Hosp. Dermatol. Soc.*; **56**: 79–99.

Crow, KD and Puhvel, SM (1991), Chloracne (halogen acne), *Dermatotoxicology*, Hemisphere, New York, 647–65.

Kokelj, F (1992), Occupational acne, *Clinics in Dermatol.*; **10**: 213–17.

Moses, M and Prioleau, PG (1985), Cutaneous histological findings in chemical workers with and without past exposure to 2,3,7,8-tetrachlorodibenzo-*p*-dioxin, *J. Am. Acad. Dermatol.*; **12**: 497–506.

Sperling, L (1994), Skin diseases associated with excessive heat, humidity, and sunlight, *Textbook of Military Medicine* (Part III), Office of the Surgeon General, Department of the Army, Falls Church, VA, 44–5.

Taylor, JS (1979), Environmental chloracne: update and review, *Annals NY Acad. of Sciences*; **320**: 295–307.

Tindall, JP (1985), Chloracne and chloracnegens, *J. Am. Acad. Dermatol.*; **13**(4): 539–58.

CHAPTER NINE

OCCUPATIONAL SKIN CANCER

Rosemary Nixon

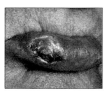

Scrotal squamous carcinoma in a machinist.

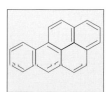

The polycyclic hydrocarbon benzo(a)pyrene.

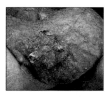

Squamous cell carcinoma of lower lip in a farmer; tobacco is a co-carcinogen with UVR.

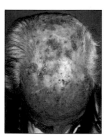

Bald outdoor workers are prone to actinic damage to the scalp.

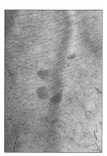

Tar warts are found in machinists who have been in contact with mineral oil for many years.

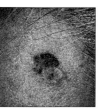

Basal cell carcinoma induced by ultraviolet radiation.

INTRODUCTION

Occupational skin cancers are defined as those where a person's occupation has played a major role in the aetiology of the tumour. Currently, multiple aetiological factors are thought to contribute to the development of skin cancer. In the past, however, there have been several virtual epidemics of skin cancer, which were traceable to occupational exposures. The major occupational carcinogens recognised were polycyclic hydrocarbons, ionising radiation and arsenic (*Tables 28, 29*).

Ultraviolet radiation is now the most important carcinogen in the aetiology of occupational skin cancer.

Table 28. Causative agents in occupational skin cancer.

Polycyclic hydrocarbons – soot; tar; pitch; mineral oil; shale oil; crude paraffin; asphalt
Ionising radiation
Arsenic
UV light

Table 29. Occupations with potential exposure to causative agents in occupational skin cancer.

Causative agent	Occupation
Polycyclic hydrocarbons	Tar distilling; coal gas manufacturing; briquettes manufacturing; shale oil workers; refinery workers
UV light	Outdoor workers; welders; laser exposure; printers
Ionising radiation	Nuclear power plant workers; radiography technicians; uranium mining

HISTORICAL REVIEW

Polycyclic hydrocarbons

Polycyclic hydrocarbons are produced by the incomplete combustion and distillation of coal, natural gas and oil shale. These chemicals are contained in tar, fuel oils, lubricating oils and greases, oil shale and bitumen.

In 1775 the first cancer of any type to be linked with occupational exposure was reported by Percivall Pott. He described the occurrence of scrotal squamous cell carcinomas (SCCs) (257) in chimney sweeps in Britain, often occurring some years after the exposure to soot and chimney dust had ceased. The scrotal carcinomas were often preceded by hyperkeratotic lesions on the scrotum known as 'soot warts'.

Henry Butlin, a surgeon, investigated scrotal cancer from 1889 to 1891 and observed that in parts of Europe the disease was unknown. In Britain sweeps

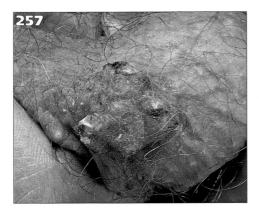

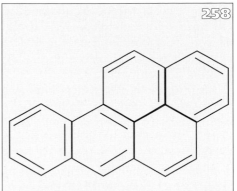

257 Scrotal squamous carcinoma in a machinist who had contact with mineral oils for many years.

258 Benzo(a)pyrene.

worked from a young age with very little protective clothing. Even as long ago as 1785, German chimney sweeps had completely covered themselves with clothing, without any possibility of skin exposure to soot; also, in Germany, wood rather than coal was used for heating. Soot formed by burning wood has much lower levels of the polycyclic hydrocarbon benzo(a)pyrene (258), implicated in the aetiology of skin cancer compared to coal soot. Skin cancer was still reported in chimney sweeps in Britain in the 1950s.

The next group of workers who appeared to have occupational skin cancer were those working with tar and pitch. Von Volkman first presented cases in Berlin in 1873 and in 1907 such cases were recognised in the British Workers Compensation Act. In 1932 Kennaway described the carcinogenic effect of 1,2,5,6-dibenzanthracene in animal models. The cancers reported after exposure to tar and pitch were similar to those observed in chimney sweeps though they tended to be located on exposed areas. The latent period was 15–25 years. By 1945 in Britain, almost 50% of industrial skin cancer was attributable to expo-

sure to pitch and tar – by 1953 there were approximately 250 cases yearly.

Shale oil had also been described as causing skin cancer, the earliest report being that by Bell in 1876. In a report in 1937 Henry described 1631 workers who died of carcinoma of the scrotum from 1911 to 1938 (257). The predominant cause was contact with shale oil which is mineral oil removed from shale by extractive distillation. This was used to produce naphtha, lubricating oil and solid paraffin. This epidemic concerned men employed in the textile industry, the so-called Lancashire Mule Spinners. In 1922 Southan described this condition, in which cancers occurred predominantly on the scrotum but also on the arms, hands and face. The mule spinners leaned over a carriage bar to twist broken threads as they wound about a spindle. The spindles were lubricated with Scottish shale oil which soaked the spinners' trousers.

Mineral oil was also recognised as being carcinogenic along with bitumen and paraffin by the British Workers Compensation Authority in 1914. Jute workers were exposed to mineral oils. Jute was treated with an emulsion of oil and water before it was spun, thus exposing the process worker to unnaturally oily fibre in addition to contact with the oil used in the lubricating machinery. The peak incidence of skin cancer caused by mineral oil occurred in 1928.

An upsurge in skin cancer amongst tool setters occurred in the light engineering industry where contact with mineral oils occurred particularly on exposed areas of the arms. Mineral oil was dripped on the spinning machine parts in order to cool them. By 1959 there were 190 cases of skin cancer attributable to tar and pitch in Britain, 20 in the cotton industry and 16 related to contact with other mineral oils (259).

A case of multiple keratoses and squamous cell carcinoma from cutting oil was reported in Japan as recently as 1992.

Another group that was occupationally exposed was wax pressmen who were involved in the production of refined wax from crude petroleum. Fractional distillation was used to separate the wax-containing distillate from the crude oil. The distillate was chilled and then pumped at high pressure into Moore wax presses. The wax was pressed out of the oil. This wax contained 20–40% of the oil distillate which was the active carcinogenic fraction. Presses were broken open to permit separation of the individual plates and slack – or crude – wax was removed manually from the plates with bars by a team of workers known as pressmen. After removal, the slack wax was dropped down a conveyor system, transferred to a receiver tank, melted and then pumped into treating plant storage tanks where it was treated. The separation and dewaxing of the plates involved leaning across the side rail to clean them. Workers' clothing became saturated with slack wax usually in the lower abdominal and genital areas, especially if a pro-

tective apron was not worn. Without washing, the exposure became effectively continuous. This process was replaced in 1951 by solvent extraction.

Ionising radiation

Occupational exposure to ionising radiation was associated with development of skin cancers particularly in the early years of this century. Doctors, dentists, nurses and technicians were exposed to radiation, particularly on the hands exposed during radiotherapy treatments. The development of squamous cell carcinoma was usually preceded by radiodermatitis or ulceration. With the advent of appropriate protective equipment by the 1930s such lesions were seldom seen. However, occupational sources of ionising radiation exist today in areas such as nuclear power plants, medical investigations and uranium mining (260).

Arsenic

Systemic arsenic absorption is associated with the development of pathognomonic skin changes including punctate keratoses, pigmentary changes and skin cancer; the vast majority of these cases were associated with ingestion, when arsenic has been used either for medicinal purposes or had contaminated drinking water. Even in 1947 it was commented that the total number of occupational cases was astonishingly small in comparison with the large number of people exposed to arsenic in industry. Most cases of arsenic ingestion or inhalation contributing to skin cancer were described in those exposed to arsenic dust in mining and smelting, those working with sheep dip and people handling insecticides and pesticides such as vintners, gardeners, nurserymen and seedsmen (261). These cases dated to the

259 Pigmented tar keratoses.

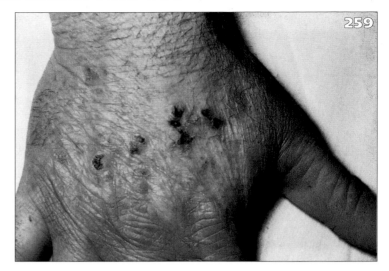

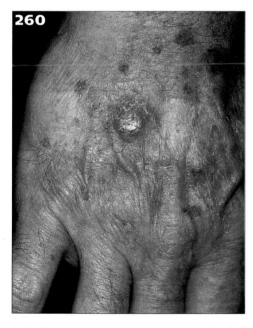

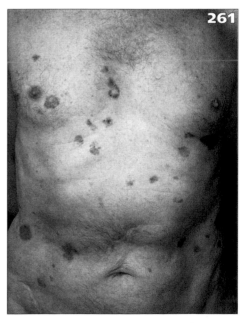

260 Squamous cell carcinoma on the back of the hand of a soldier who had observed nuclear weapons tests.

261 Multiple BCC following arsenic ingestion.

1930s and as work conditions improved fewer cases were reported.

Ultraviolet (UV) light

The association of excessive sunlight exposure with the development of skin cancers has been credited to Unna who described the changes on the skin of sailors. Subsequently there have been multiple attempts to identify risk factors both for non-melanocytic skin cancer comprising basal cell carcinomas (BCCs), squamous cell carcinomas (SCCs) and malignant melanomas. There is general agreement that tumours arise because of the combination of certain host factors and certain environmental factors. In SCC, for example, the host risk factors include older age, male sex, skin that tans poorly, skin that burns easily after sunlight exposure,

freckling, Celtic ancestry, fair skin, red, blond or light brown hair and blue or light-coloured eyes. People with a genetic susceptibility such as xeroderma pigmentosum (262) or with a chronic scarring condition are also more prone to develop SCC.

Environmental factors thought to be relevant include sunlight exposure as indicated by latitude of residence, and occupational or recreational exposure. Other sources of UV light may include artificial tanning and photochemotherapy. Other factors include ionising radiation, cigarette smoking for SCC of the lip (263) and other relevant occupational exposures such as that to polycyclic hydrocarbons; UV light may act as a promoter in the development of skin tumours from polycyclic hydrocarbons.

There is certainly controversy about the role of UV light, particularly in the

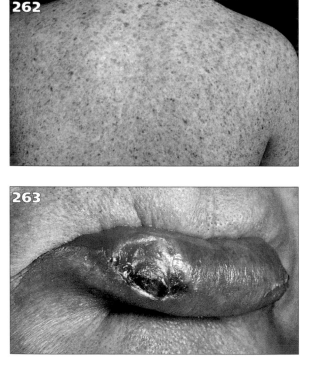

262 Xeroderma pigmentosa.

263 SCC of the lower lip in a farmer.

aetiology of BCCs and malignant melanomas. These tumours are much more likely to be found on non-sunlight-exposed sites more often than SCCs. Childhood sunlight exposure is thought to be important in the aetiology of both tumours and, in particular, for malignant melanoma; intermittent intensive sunlight exposure such as with sunburn is thought to be important. On the other hand, cumulative exposure seems to be most relevant in the causation of SCCs. Some of this information is quite difficult to prove epidemiologically because of the effects of recall bias and the difficulties in estimating lifetime occupational and recreational sunlight exposure.

DIAGNOSIS

The diagnosis of occupational skin cancer is similar to that of the non-occupational type in that generally the exposed sites are involved. Previously the scrotum was involved frequently because of continuous exposure to carcinogens and the increased likelihood of skin absorption in that site (see **257**).

There may be co-existing signs of exposure prior to – or in addition to – evidence of skin cancer. These may include oil folliculitis and hyperkeratoses described in people working with mineral oil, and pitch or tar warts. Oil hyperkeratoses were described as being flat, white, circular, hyperkeratotic smooth plaques, small in diameter and often clustered. There were also verrucose pigmented round or oval irregular raised warts. Tar warts were pigmented small papules which were often seen around the face on the eyes, eyelids, cheek, forearms and back of the hands (**264, 265**).

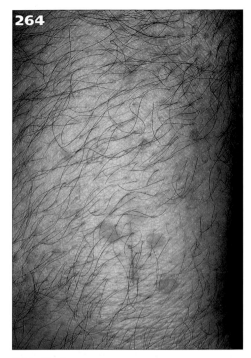

264 Tar keratoses.

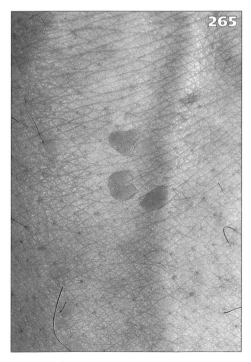

265 Tar keratoses.

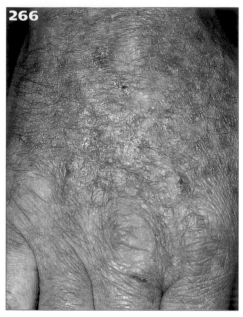

266 Solar keratoses.

Solar keratoses (**266**, **267**) caused by actinic exposure tend to be red, scaly and sometimes pigmented and are found on sunlight exposed areas such as the backs of the hands and the face. BCCs can be of a number of types but are most commonly nodulo-ulcerative – the majority of these occur on the face. They are often raised, pearly and cystic with superficial telangiectases; there is often a history of bleeding and ulceration (**268–270**). On the other hand, superficial BCCs are often found on the trunk. These are red, flat or only very slightly raised, scaly and may vary in diameter (**271**).

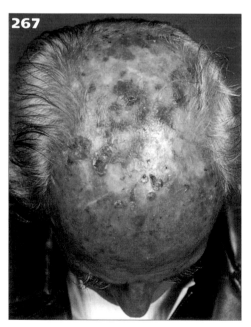

267 Solar keratoses.

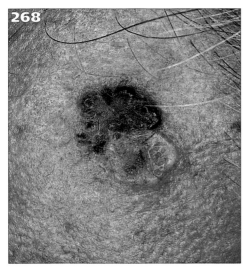

268 Pigmented BCC.

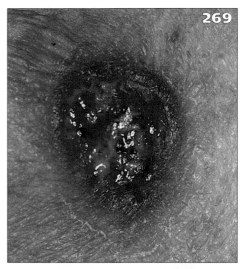

269 Ulcerating nodular cystic BCC.

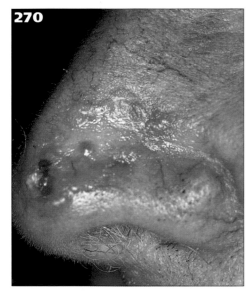

270 Morphoeic BCC on the nose.

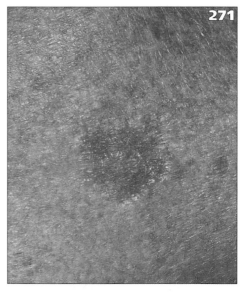

271 Superficial BCC on the shoulder of a professional yachtsman.

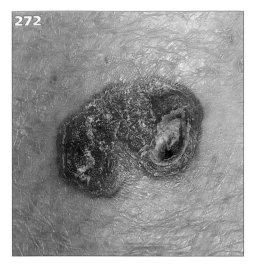

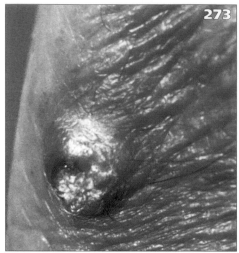

272 Bowens – intra-epidermal SCC.

273 SCC on the back of the hand of road builder.

SCCs are commonly found on sunlight exposed sites such as the back of the hands and the face (**272–274**). These are often firm, tender, scaly nodules; ulceration may occasionally occur. They are prone to occur on the more sunlight exposed lower lip in people with a history of such exposure. Cigarette smoking is probably a co-carcinogen for lip SCC.

SCCs are thought to metastasise at the rate of approximately 2% but lesions on the lip and ear metastasise at a greater rate of approximately 10%.

Malignant melanomas are usually one of the following types:

- Lentigo maligna melanomas (**275**) are commonly found in the sunlight exposed areas of the face and often arise in long-standing lesions known as lentigo maligna (Hutchinson's melanotic freckle). These tend to be associated with a cumulative history of sunlight exposure.

- Superficial spreading melanomas – which are less related to sunlight exposure – commonly occur on the legs in women (**276**) and on the back in men. They are irregular pigmented, often black and, in early stages, are quite flat. They may, however, have an irregular edge or irregular distribution of pigmentation. They are usually more than 6 mm in diameter (**277**).

- Nodular melanomas (**278**) – also less related to sunlight exposure – often arise quickly as black papules or nodules which often tend to ulcerate and bleed. Because their growth rate is rapid the prognosis is generally much worse at presentation than compared with superficial spreading melanomas.

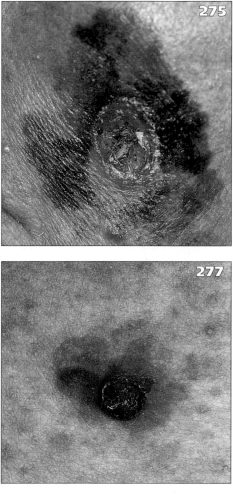

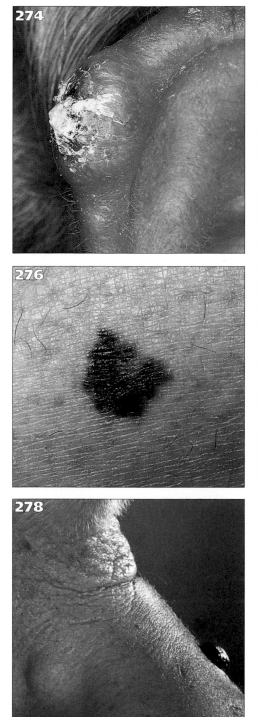

274 SCC of the ear-lobe of a farmer.

275 Lentigo maligna melanoma.

276 Early (good prognosis) superficial spreading melanoma on the leg of an air hostess.

277 A nodule in a superficial malignant melanoma. Breslow thickness was 2.3 mm.

278 Nodular melanoma with regional lymphadenopathy (poor prognosis).

MANAGEMENT

Prevention of the development of skin cancers is most important. In the workplace it is important to consider substitution of carcinogens where possible – this has certainly been done with declining exposure to polycyclic hydrocarbons in recent decades. Protection of the skin, with either protective clothing or engineering control such as machine guarding is important. Daily washing is essential. Since most of the skin cancers are associated with a very long latency period, it is important to have continued surveillance of older or retired workers.

Finally, the skin cancers need to be treated as appropriate. Generally, removal by excision is favoured to ensure complete histological examination and identification of the uninvolved tissue margin. However, other possible measures include curettage and diathermy for BCCs, appropriately controlled cryotherapy for SCCs and radiotherapy. It is recommended that suspected malignant melanomas be excised with a 2 mm margin, a later decision being made on any appropriate re-excision margins. In some cases, elective lymph node dissection is performed but this remains controversial. Results of treatments for metastatic melanoma are only fair and include isolated limb perfusion, chemotherapy and immunotherapy.

BIBLIOGRAPHY

Armstrong, BK (1988), Epidemiology of malignant melanoma; intermittent or total accumulated exposure to the sun, *J. Dermatol. Surg. Oncol.*; **14**: 835–49.

Blum, H (1945), Sunlight is a causal factor in cancer of the skin in man, *J. Nat. Cancer Inst.*; **9**: 247–58.

Cruikshank, CD and Squire, JR (1950), Skin cancer in the engineering industry from the use of mineral oil, *Br. J. Indust. Med.*; 7: 1–11.

Emmett, EA (1975), Occupational skin cancer; a review, *J. Occup. Med.*; **17**: 44–9.

Epstein, JH, Ormsby, A and Adams, RM (1990), Occupational skin cancer, *Occupational Skin Disease*, W.B. Saunders Co., Philadelphia, 136.

Fife, JG (1962), Carcinoma of the skin in machine tool setters, *Br. J. Indust. Med.*; **19**: 123–5.

Kinnear, J, Rogers, J, Finn, OA and Nair, A (1955), Dermatoses in jute workers, *Br. J. Indust. Med.*; **12**: 36–42.

Kricker, A, Armstrong, BK and English, DR (1994), Sun exposure and non-melanocytic skin cancer, *Cancer Causes and Control*; **5**: 367–92.

Lione, JG, Denholme, JS (1959) Cancer of the scrotum in wax pressmen, *AMA Arch. Indust. Health*; **19**: 530–9.

Neubauer, O (1947), Arsenical cancer, a review, *Br. J. Cancer*; **1**: 192–251.

Tsuji, T, Otake, N, Kobayashi, T and Miwa, N (1992), Multiple keratoses and squamous cell carcinoma from cutting oil, *J. Am. Acad. Derm.*; **27**: 767–8.

Waldron, HA (1983), A brief history of scrotal cancer, *Br. J. Indust. Med.*; **40**: 390–401.

CHAPTER TEN

PIGMENTARY CHANGES RELATED TO OCCUPATION

David J Gawkrodger

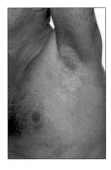

Sites not exposed directly to the depigmenting chemical can be affected.

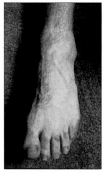

Occupational leukoderma.

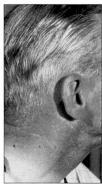

Argyria usually affects exposed areas.

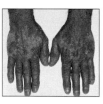

Symmetrical occupational leukoderma.

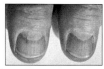

The nails can show a bluish discoloration in argyria.

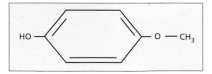

Monomethylether of hydroquinone is a substituted phenolic compound.

OCCUPATIONAL LEUKODERMA (OCCUPATIONAL 'VITILIGO')

Definition

Occupational leukoderma is defined as pigmentation or hypopigmentation of the skin due to industrial exposure to a chemical or chemicals known to have a destructive effect on epidermal melanocytes (**279**). Post-inflammatory hypopigmentation – resulting from chemical, thermal, radiation or traumatic scarring, or following a straightforward allergic contact dermatitis reaction – are excluded from discussion in this section.

Historical review

Depigmentation due to a chemical was first reported in 1939 when tannery workers in Chicago were found to have depigmentation of the skin on their forearms and the dorsal aspects of their hands. In some workers other parts of the body were affected.

The operators thought that rubber gloves were to blame and it was discovered that monobenzylether of hydroquinone was responsible. This had been used in the manufacture of the rubber

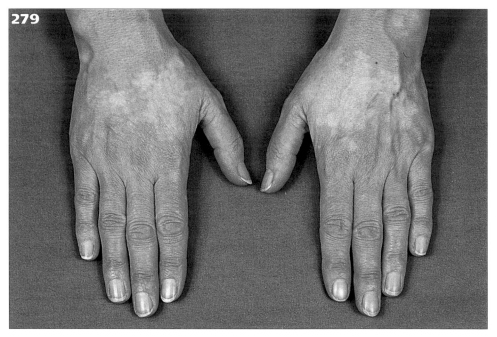

279 Vitiligo – was it occupational? Clinically it is very difficult to distinguish between idiopathic and occupational leukoderma.

gloves to make them more durable. After this chemical was removed from the rubber gloves, repigmentation occurred in some workers after a few months, and within 3 years all had regained their normal skin colour. Following this, other cases of depigmentation due to rubber contact in tannery workers were reported and monobenzylether of hydroquinone was removed from rubber. Nonetheless, hypopigmentation from this chemical is still seen as it is sometimes used therapeutically to induce leukoderma. In addition to its toxic effect on melanocytes it is also a sensitiser.

Chemicals causing occupational vitiligo

Certain chemicals, particularly the substituted phenols (280, 281), are destructive to functional melanocytes. Many of these compounds cause permanent depigmentation of the skin such as that seen in vitiligo. The chemicals most commonly responsible for this are:

- *p*-Tertiary butylphenol (282).
- *p*-Tertiary butylcatechol (283).
- Monobenzylether of hydroquinone.
- Hydroquinone (and related compounds).

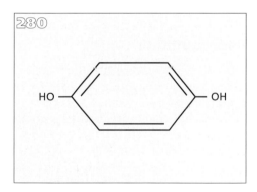

280 Hydroquinone.

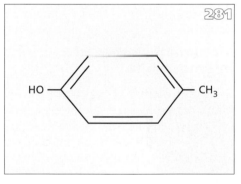

281 *p*-Cresol.

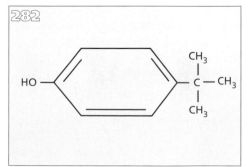

282 *p*-Tertiary butylphenol.

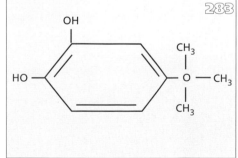

283 *p*-Tertiary butylcatechol.

149

Table 30. Chemicals capable of causing occupational leukoderma.

Hydroquinone
Monobenzylether of hydroquinone
Monoethylether of hydroquinone (*p*-ethoxyphenol)
Monomethylether of hydroquinone (*p*-methoxyphenol)
p-cresol
p-isopropylcatechol
p-methylcatechol
p-nonylphenol
p-octylphenol
p-phenylphenol
p-tertiary amylphenol
p-tertiary butylcatechol
p-tertiary butylphenol
N,N',N''-triethylenethiophosphoramide (thio-TEPA)
Mercaptoamines, e.g. *N*-2-mercaptoethyldimethylamine hydrochloride (MEDA)
Physostigmine

A list of chemicals known to cause occupational leukoderma is shown in *Table 30*.

Monomethylether of hydroquinone

Monomethylether of hydroquinone (4-hydroxyanisole or 4-methoxyphenol, 284) is an intermediate in the manufacture of several chemicals. It is also used as a stabiliser for chlorinated hydrocarbons and ethylcellulose and as a polymerisation inhibitor for acrylic monomers. Occupational leukoderma due to exposure to monomethylether of hydroquinone has been reported when it

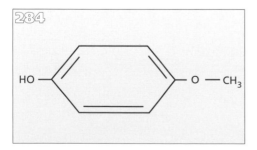

284 Monomethylether of hydroquinone.

was used as a stabiliser for the manufacture of vinylidene chloride.

Hydroquinone

Hydroquinone can also induce leukoderma although its effect and potency as a contact allergen is not so great as monobenzylether of hydroquinone. Hydroquinone rarely produces complete depigmentation but it can result in hypopigmentation. Hydroquinone is used in photographic developing.

p-Cresol

p-Cresol can result in leukoderma. It is a chemical with many uses including disinfectant, textile scouring agent, food flavouring, and in the manufacture of phenolic compounds.

p-Tertiary butylphenol

p-Tertiary butylphenol was recognised as causing leukoderma in the 1960s although it had been previously recognised as a contact sensitiser. Leukoderma was reported in workers involved in the manufacture of *p*-tertiary butylphenol formaldehyde resin. In the late 1960s occupational leukoderma due to this compound was described in workers in the shoe industry.

Depigmentation due to substituted phenols used in a cleaning fluid was described in the 1970s. *p*-Tertiary butylphenol, *p*-tertiary amylphenol, *o*-phenylphenol and *o*-benzyl-*p*-chlorophenol were present in the fluid. Affected individuals had depigmentation at distant sites as well as at points of contact. Occupational leukoderma was reported in 54 of 198 persons involved in the manufacture of *p*-tertiary butylphenol.

Para-tertiary butylcatechol

p-Tertiary butylcatechol is another agent that can cause leukoderma. Four of 75 workers exposed to this compound (added as an anti-oxidant to an oil used in the assembly of tappets) developed leukoderma. Not only did they have local depigmentation on the hands and arms but distant sites were affected in three out of the four; patch tests were positive in three of the four subjects. Occupational leukoderma with associated contact sensitivity has also been described in an individual who was employed as a batteryman and labourer at a coke works, where he had contact with coal tar and tar products.

Clinical features

Idiopathic vitiligo is much more common than occupationally induced leukoderma although often the two cannot be differentiated on the basis of the clinical pattern of the disease. Idiopathic vitiligo affects 1–2% of the general population, usually presenting with a symmetrical pattern of depigmentation over the dorsal aspects of the hands and forearms, around the mouth or eyes, or on the trunk. It starts typically in the second

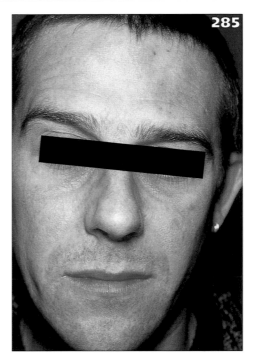

285 Leukoderma of the face due to occupational contact with *p*-tertiary butylphenol.

decade, shows a family history of 30% of cases and may be associated with autoantibodies to thyroid or other tissues.

In some individuals with occupational vitiligo, the leukoderma has been confined to the parts of the body exposed to the chemical, usually the hands and forearms (285–289).

However, in many reported cases, the depigmentation has been more extensive and away from areas of skin in which direct contact would be expected. This has given rise to the suggestion that the depigmentation is due to systemic exposure to the chemical, either by percutaneous absorption, inhalation or ingestion. In support of this is the observation that some workers with occupational leukoderma due to *p*-tertiary butylphenol have also had abnormal liver function tests.

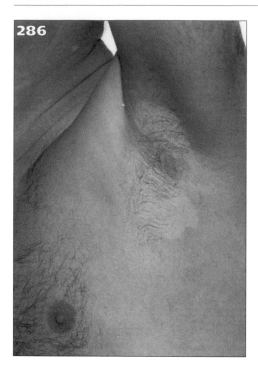

286 Axillary leukoderma caused by occupational exposure to *p*-tertiary butylphenol.

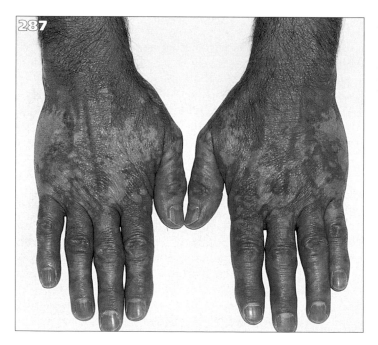

287 Symmetrical leukoderma of the dorsal aspects of the hands due to occupational contact with hydroquinone.

288 Symmetrical leukoderma of the wrists following occupational contact with hydroquinone.

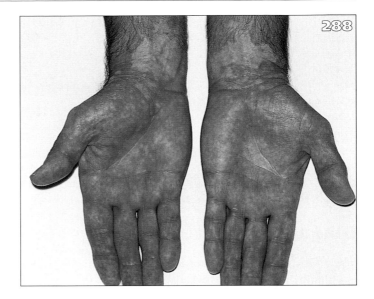

289 Leukoderma on the foot due to exposure to *p*-tertiary butylphenol in a worker manufacturing phenolic resins for the car industry.

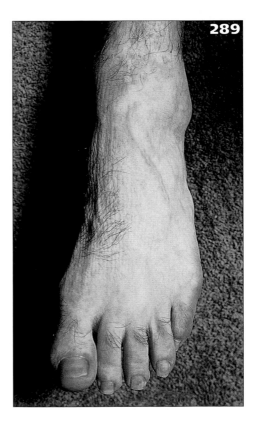

In some cases there is a history of antecedent or concurrent allergic contact dermatitis from the offending chemicals. The minimum time for skin depigmentation to develop is 2–4 weeks. Laboratory studies suggest that pigment loss through repeated contact with chemicals may take 6 months to become visible although, of several workers with apparently the same level of exposure to a chemical, only a minority will develop occupational leukoderma. The reason for this is not known.

Diagnosis

The diagnosis of occupational vitiligo should be suspected if a worker who has been potentially exposed to depigmenting chemicals develops leukoderma on the dorsal aspects of the hands or in a more widespread distribution. There should be particular suspicion if more than one worker is involved. The chemicals to which the worker is exposed should be identified and investigation made to see if it or they are known to cause depigmentation.

Some occupations known to be at risk of exposure to depigmenting chemicals are shown in *Table 31*.

Patch testing is indicated to investigate whether there is coexisting contact sensitivity to the chemical. This may be found with *p*-tertiary butylcatechol although it is not a prerequisite for the diagnosis of occupational vitiligo.

Mechanisms of depigmentation

The depigmentary effect of the phenolic compounds is thought to be by a toxic mechanism on the melanocyte (**290**, **291**). It is proposed that the chemical requirement for depigmentation is the hydroxyl group in the *para* (4) position with a non-polar side group in the 1 position. Alkyl phenols are chemically similar to tyrosine (**292**) and may be oxidised by tyrosinase to give rise to a free radical derivative which is highly toxic to the melanocyte.

Management

There is no specific treatment for occupational vitiligo. Removal of the offending chemical may result in partial repigmentation but this process may take years and may even not occur at all. Treatment should be aimed at preventing further exposure. Camouflage cosmetics may be used and the depigmented skin protected from UV irradiation by sunscreens.

Table 31. Occupations with potential exposure to depigmenting chemicals.

Manufacture of or exposure to:

Insecticides; paints; plastics; rubber
Lubricating and motor oils
Photographic chemicals
Antimicrobials and disinfectants
Detergents and deodorants
Inks

290 Melanocytes in normal skin, as demonstrated by DOPA staining.

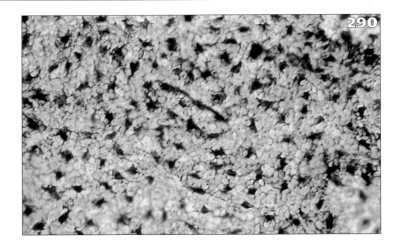

291 A considerable reduction in the numbers of melanocytes in skin affected by occupational leukoderma, as demonstrated by DOPA staining.

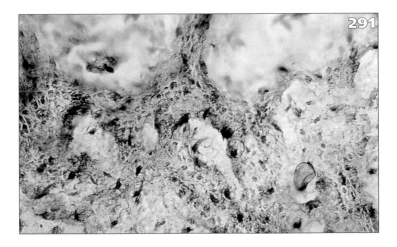

292 Tyrosine.

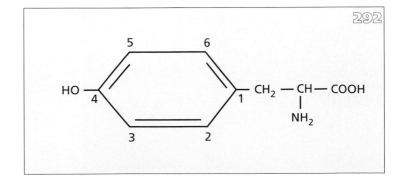

ARGYRIA

Silver may be deposited in the skin from industrial exposure to silver salts or silver fumes (**293, 294**). The pigmentation is usually slatey-grey in colour and mainly occurs in sun-exposed sites, especially the face and hands (**295, 296**). It may be clinically apparent within a few months of exposure but more usually it takes several years for the skin discoloration to appear depending on the degree of exposure. In some people the entire skin assumes a slatey-blue/grey hue.

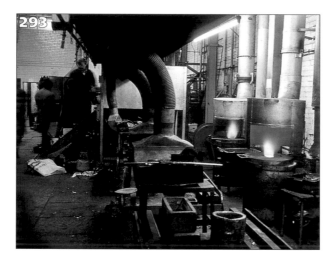

293 A workshop in which silver is being refined into silver ingots. Furnaces and extraction hoods to remove the fumes are evident.

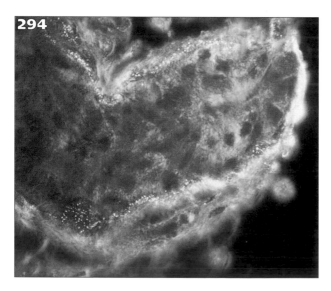

294 Skin biopsy is a useful method of establishing the diagnosis of argyria. Granules of silver are deposited in the basement membrane of eccrine sweat glands and are demonstrated by the use of polarised light. They may also be shown by electron microscopy. X-ray dispersive microanalysis confirms that the granules contain silver. In fact the silver is widely distributed in tissues other than the skin.

295 Argyria, showing slatey-grey pigmentation of the neck in a silver refiner. The pigmentation is permanent. Treatment with depigmenting preparations is unsuccessful.

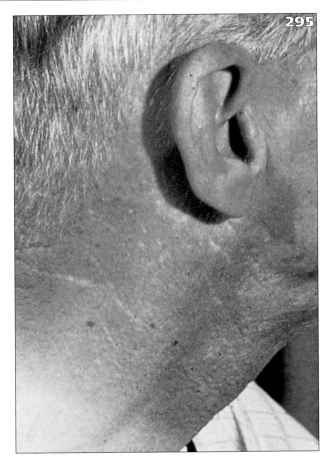

296 The nails may show a bluish discoloration in argyria. The sclerae and mucous membranes can also show the same changes in colour.

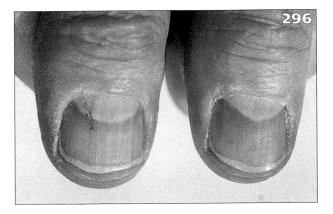

Table 32. Changes in skin colour due to chemical occupational exposure.

Colour	Chemical	Occupation	Comment
Blue/grey	Osmium trioxide	Lab. technicians; lamp makers; chemical manufacturers, platinum hardeners	Black skin pigmentation
	Silver/silver salts	Silver platers; photographic developers	Argyria: slate-grey pigment seen on sun-exposed sites; permanent
Brown	*p*-Phenylenediamine	Dye makers; photo graphic developers	Stains skin
	Permanganates	Bleach/dye makers; water purifiers; paper makers	Stains skin
	Phenothiazine	Farmers; vets; nurses	Phenothiazine– melanin complexes deposited in skin
Green	Copper dust	Electrical workers; machinists; copper smelters	Greenish-black dis-coloration of hair, skin and teeth
Yellow	Anthracene	Tar distillation	Stains skin; photo-sensitiser
	Fluorescein dye Glutaraldehyde	Manufacture Laboratory; medical; dentistry; leather tanning; embalming	Photosensitiser, stains skin
	Picric acid/picrates Trinitrotoluene (TNT)	Dye industry; explosives Explosives	Transient staining Transient staining

OTHER CHANGES IN SKIN PIGMENTATION RELATED TO OCCUPATION

Some chemicals can stain or be absorbed and cause changes in skin colour. Details are given in *Table 32*.

ACKNOWLEDGEMENT

I am very grateful to Professor S.S. Bleehen, Dr C.J. Stevenson, Dr C.I. Harrington and Dr J.S.C. English for advice in the preparation of this text and for allowing me to reproduce some of their figures.

BIBLIOGRAPHY

Bleehen, SS, Gould, DJ, Harrington, CI *et al.* (1981), Occupational argyria: light and electron microscopic studies and X-ray micro-analysis, *Br. J. Dermatol.*; **104**: 19–26.

Calnan, CD and Cooke, MA (1974), Leukoderma in industry, *J. Soc. Occup. Med.*; **24**: 59–61.

Gawkrodger, DJ, Cork, MJ and Bleehen, SS (1991), Occupational vitiligo and contact sensitivity to paratertiary butyl catechol, *Contact Dermatitis*; **25**: 200–1.

Kahn, G (1970), Depigmentation caused by phenolic detergents, *Arch. Dermatol.*; **102**: 177–80.

CHAPTER ELEVEN

OCCUPATIONAL CONNECTIVE TISSUE DISORDERS

Volker Ziegler

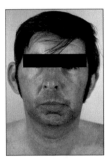

Bone resorption of the jaw in vinyl chloride disease.

Pulmonary fibrosis due to silicosis.

Acrosclerosis with rat-bite necrosis.

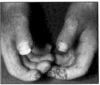

Finger contractures in systemic sclerosis.

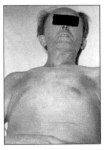

Terminal systemic sclerosis.

Raynaud's phenomenon.

SCLERODERMA

Scleroderma is a relatively rare connective tissue disease which can affect the skin and internal organs. The incidence is approximately 10 cases per million of the general population and the prevalence varies considerably between 50 and 100 cases per million. Women are affected three to six times more frequently than men. The principal patho-logical changes are abnormalities of the immune and circulatory systems as well as changes in the composition of collagen. The aetiology of a proportion of cases can be related to environmental and occupational substances. Clinically the so-called scleroderma-like illness can be distinguished from systemic sclerosis and morphoea.

SCLERODERMA-LIKE DISEASE

Scleroderma-like diseases have been observed increasingly over the past 20 years. These comprise diseases that, in addition to skin changes similar to those of scleroderma, also involve other organ systems, but are not consistent with classic scleroderma. The most important aetiological factors and clinical manifestations are summarised in *Table 33*.

A common factor in these diseases is that they generally show definite clinical improvement when exposure to the relevant agent ceases (apart from silicon-induced systemic sclerosis).

Vinyl chloride disease

Up to 6% of operatives working in the manufacture of polyvinyl chloride (PVC), especially reactor cleaners, develop changes mainly on the hands, forearms, feet and face. Parotitis, hepatomegaly, splenomegaly and bone resorption are also seen (**297, 298**). Thrombocytopenia and non-organ specific auotantibodies are recognised to occur in this disease. The prognosis is unknown but angiosarcoma of the liver is a fatal complication.

Vinyl chloride – CH_2CHCl – when polymerised produces PVC. Exposure levels to the monomer should not exceed 5 parts per million.

Table 33. Scleroderma-like diseases related to occupational and environmental factors.

Inducing factors	Symptoms
Occupational agents	
Vinyl chloride	Raynaud's phenomenon; sclerodactyly; acro-osteolysis; hepatic fibrosis; angiosarcoma; plaque-like fibrotic cutaneous lesions; leuco- and thrombocytopenia
Organic solvents	Skin fibrosis; irritant dermatitis; hepatitis; neurological symptoms
Bis(4-amino-3-methyl-cyclohexyl)methane – for epoxy production	Skin sclerosis; erythema; fatigue; myalgia; arthralgia
Iatrogenic agents	
Bleomycin	Pulmonary fibrosis; scleroderma-like lesions
Pentazocine	Pigmentary changes; panniculitis; ulcerations and sclerotic fibrosis on injection sites
L-tryptophan	Sclerodermatous induration; peripheral eosinophilia; myalgia; arthralgia
Silicon	Systemic sclerosis; Sjögren's syndrome; arthritis
Other substances	
Toxic oil syndrome	Scleroderma-like changes; neuromuscular atrophy; hypertension; Sicca syndrome

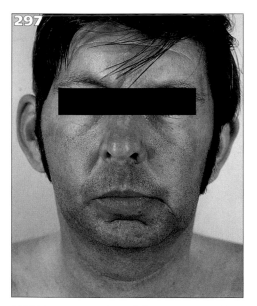

297 Bone resorption of the jaw in a PVC manufacturing process operative.

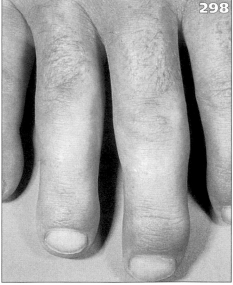

298 The same patient's hands showing acrosclerosis with marked resorption of bone at the distal phalanges.

161

QUARTZ-INDUCED SCLERODERMA

Epidemiological and occupational medicine aspects

Quartz (silicon dioxide; SiO_2) is widely distributed in nature (**299**). Silicon-derived materials (predominantly as quartz) account for 27% of the Earth's

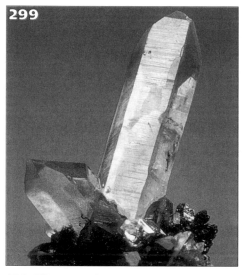

299 Silica crystals.

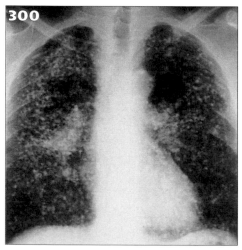

300 Silicosis of the lungs.

crust. Silicon dioxide is present in over 90% of all minerals; it is chemically virtually inactive and can remain unaltered for decades in human tissues. Its principle medical significance is as the causative agent of pulmonary silicosis (**300**).

The first suggestion of a possible association between occupational exposure and the development of systemic sclerosis came from the Scottish physician Bramwell (1914). He observed nine patients of whom five had worked as stonemasons. Erasmus (1957) reported 16 cases of scleroderma amongst 8000 miners in South African gold mines, in comparison to a control group of 25 000 hospital patients without a single case of scleroderma. Since then similar case reports and studies have been published in the USA, France, Italy, Japan, Switzerland, Canada and Germany.

The most extensive results originated in the former German Democratic Republic. In 1979–80 a cross-sectional survey from the eastern part of present-day Germany reported 189 cases of scleroderma – 43 of these patients were male and of these 23 had had definite occupational exposure to quartz and ten also had coexisting silicosis. This gives rise to an odds ratio of 35:1 for men exposed to quartz; this approximates to the relative risk of developing bronchial carcinoma for a heavy smoker. This association was not seen in women as they rarely engage in occupations involving exposure to quartz.

Until 1992 a total of 125 male scleroderma patients had been registered in the Leipzig Skin Clinic, of whom 101

Table 34. Occupations of 101 male and three female scleroderma patients with a history of quartz exposure.

Occupation	Number
Miner (underground)	75
Foundry worker/cast-polisher	9
Quarry worker	6
Sandblaster	5
Dental technician (female)	3
Oven builder	2
Sandstone sculptor	2
Glass polisher	2

(81%) had been exposed to quartz and 50 (40%) also suffered from silicosis. Only 10% of an age- and sex-matched control population of 350 had been exposed to quartz and no cases of silicosis were identified. These results show highly significant statistical associations between quartz exposure and scleroderma as well as between silicosis and scleroderma. The occupations are summarised in *Table 34*.

In 1994 comparable figures were also published from the western part of Germany: 85% of 58 male scleroderma patients had also been exposed to quartz. The relative risk of developing scleroderma for this group was approximately 1 in 120.

Quartz exposure occurs particularly in the following industries and occupations: mining; stone industry; slate industry; foundry work; fire-clay manufacture and processing; construction; rubber industry (talc is heavily contaminated with silicon dioxide); and the ceramic and glass industries.

In the medical professions there is a quartz hazard for dental technicians. In many other occupations there is unsuspected exposure to quartz which is often only detected through occupational medical analysis. Recently, scleroderma-like illness has also been described following silicone breast implants. It seems possible that these cases are similarly attributable to the quartz component of the silicon.

Clinical and pathological aspects

Clinically, progressive scleroderma is a systemic illness that affects both skin and internal organs. Typical clinical appearances are shown in **301–308**. All the illustrations are of quartz-exposed men in whom an occupational disease was recognised and who were patients of the Leipzig University Skin Clinic. The principal clinical manifestations are presented in *Table 35*.

Table 35. Clinical manifestations and pathological abnormalities in progressive scleroderma.

Skin	Internal organs
Cutaneous atrophy	Raynaud's phenomenon
Pigmentary loss	Arthralgia/arthritis
'Rat bite necrosis'	Gastrointestinal motility
Calcinosis cutis	Disturbances and stenoses
Microstomia	Achylia
Telangiectasia	Dysphonia
Acrosclerosis	Pulmonary fibrosis
Diffuse generalised scleroderma	Myocardial fibrosis; nephrosclerosis; infertility

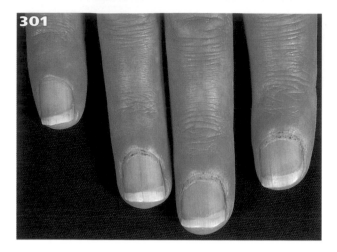

301 Nailfold infarcts in a foundry worker.

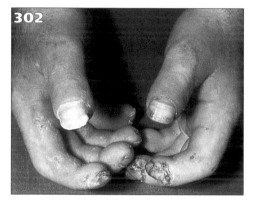

302 Systemic sclerosis with finger contractures.

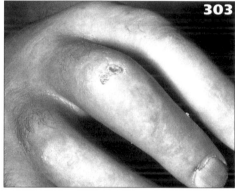

303 Acrosclerosis with rat-bite necrosis.

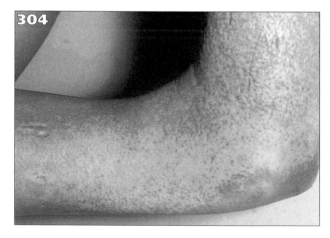

304 Diffuse scleroderma with elbow contracture.

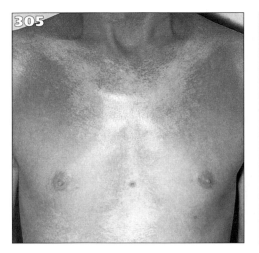

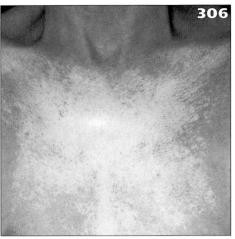

305 Diffuse systemic sclerosis with hypopigmentation.

306 Diffuse systemic sclerosis with poikilodermatous changes.

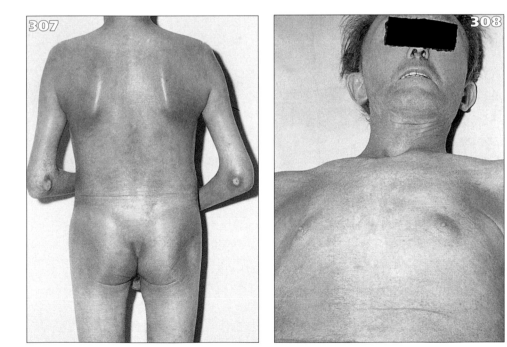

307 Diffuse systemic sclerosis with atrophy and calcinosis.

308 Pre-terminal stage of systemic sclerosis.

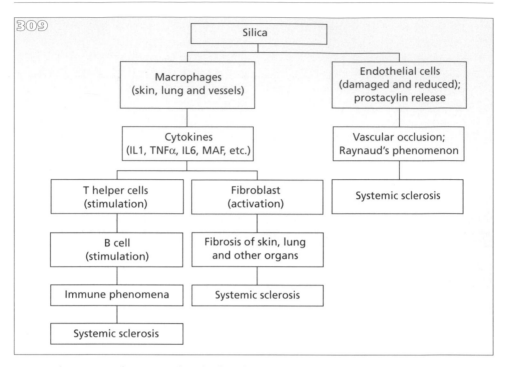

309 Pathogenesis of quartz-induced scleroderma.

American Rheumatism Association: diagnostic criteria

- Major criteria – proximal sclerosis (i.e. above the hands).
- Minor criteria – sclerodactyly; necrosis of the fingertips; basal pulmonary fibrosis; Raynaud's phenomenon.

Systemic sclerosis can be diagnosed on the finding of one major criterion and one minor criterion, or more than two minor criteria.

Treatment of scleroderma is unsatisfactory as there is no specific therapy and the course is almost always progressive. Death usually results from general debility or from renal, myocardial or pulmonary sclerosis. In cases related to the

quartz industry, removal of the patient from exposure does not result in clinical improvement. The pathogenesis of occupational scleroderma is well established as a result of intensive investigation (**309**).

Pathogenesis

Quartz can enter the body via the lungs as well as via the skin; its presence is demonstrable in both organs. Depending on the concentration present it can either have a cytotoxic effect or can induce cutaneous, alveolar and perivascular macrophages to amplify their release of cytokines (e.g. IL-1; TNF-α; MAF). These cytokines stimulate fibroblasts as well as T helper cells. B cell stimulation results in the production of the various antibodies which characterise scleroderma. The fibroblast activation leads to fibrosis of the skin, lungs and other organs. Quartz can cause Raynaud's phenomenon and vascular occlusion, possibly via damage to endothelial cells and reduced release of prostacyclin. All three pathogenic processes (immune, fibroblastic and circulatory disturbances) lead to the full clinical picture of progressive systemic sclerosis. All these processes continue to be stimulated by quartz over the years as it persists in the tissues and is virtually never eliminated. Phagocytosed quartz is liberated sooner or later by macrophages, only to be taken up again by other macrophages. Clearly other cellular systems or cytokines may be involved in this complex process. These do not, however, appear to alter the progress of the illness.

MORPHOEA

Literature on the occupational aspects of localised scleroderma, i.e. morphoea, is sparse. There is a report of generalised morphoea-like symptoms in men working with organic solvents. A recent thesis from the University of Leipzig demonstrated a statistically significant link between silica and morphoea.

LUPUS ERYTHEMATOSUS

Sunlight is an accepted exogenous factor in exacerbating as well as inducing lupus erythematosus (LE). No occupational influences were, however, demonstrated in a study of 263 patients by Nebe and Lenz. Additionally, a change from outdoor to indoor work had no significant influence on the course of the illness; a connection with silicosis has been repeatedly described.

In ex-East Germany, until 1990, all diagnoses of hospital patients were registered centrally. An evaluation of LE cases from 1985–1988 showed that one in every 61 patients also had silicosis. The population prevalence of silicosis was, however, only one in 205 males. It was found that 30 out of 64 LE patients had had occupational exposure to quartz, with 24 having systemic LE and six cutaneous LE. The affected patients were predominantly miners and foundry workers. The average duration of exposure was 11 years which is similar to that seen in scleroderma. In a study of uranium miners, a total of 37 LE patients were found of whom 30 also had silicosis. Similar cases of quartz-induced LE have been reported from Japan.

The pathogenic role of quartz could be explained by its immunostimulatory action involving secondary activation of B cells. The reported series do not, however, provide an adequate basis for a definitive conclusion and it would appear worthwhile to pursue this line of investigation.

VIBRATION WHITE FINGER

Raynaud's phenomena caused by vibrating machinery has been known for many years. In 1911 Lorigo reported vascular spasm of the fingers of miners working

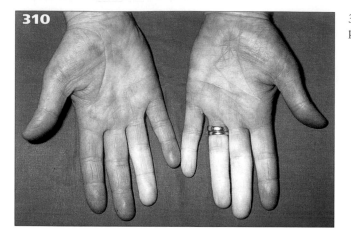

310 Idiopathic Raynaud's phenomenon.

with pneumatic tools. Idiopathic Raynaud's phenomenon tends to affect both hands (310) whereas vibration white finger may be asymmetrical.

DERMATOMYOSITIS

No occupational factors are recognised as causing dermatomyositis. In occasional cases an occupationally related tumour has led to secondary dermatomyositis. This can have implications from legal and insurance points of view.

BIBLIOGRAPHY

Bramwell, B (1914), Diffuse sclerodermia: its frequency; its occurrence in stonemasons; its treatment by fibrinolysin. Elevations of temperature due to fibrinolysin injections, *Edinburgh Med. J.*; **12**: 387.

Ebihara, I and Kawami, M (1985), Health hazards of mineral dust with special reference to the causation of immunopathological systemic diseases, *J. Science Labour*; **61**: 1–31.

Erasmus, LD (1957), Scleroderma in gold miners on the Witwatersrand with particular reference to pulmonary manifestations, *A. Afr. J. Lab. Clin. Med.*; **3**: 209.

Haustein, UF and Ziegler, V (1985), Environmentally induced systemic sclerosis-like disorders, *Int. J. Dermatol.*; **24**: 147–51.

Petzold, K (1994), *Untersuchungen zur Frage der ätiologischen Bedeutung von Quarz fur die Sklerodermie unter besonderer Berucksichtigung der zirkumskripten Sklerodermie*, Thesis, University of Leipzig.

Rowell, NR and Goodfield, MJD (1992), The connective tissue diseases, *Textbook of Dermatology*, Blackwell Scientific Publications, Oxford, 2236–7.

Rustin, MHA, Bull, HA, Ziegler, V et al. (1990), Silica associated systemic sclerosis is clinically, serologically and immunologically indistinguishable from idiopathic systemic sclerosis, *Br. J. Dermatol.*; **123**: 725–34.

Yamakage, A and Ishikawa, H (1992), Generalised morphoea-like scleroderma occurring in people exposed to organic solvents, *Dermatologica*; **165**: 186–93.

Ziegler, V and Haustein, UF (1992), Die progressive Sklerodermie – eine quarzinduzierte Berufskrankheit?, *Dermatol. Monatsschr.*; **178**: 34–43.

Ziegler, V, Pfeil, B and Haustein, UF (1991), Berufliche Quarzexposition – progressive Sklerodermie und Lupu erythematodes, *Z. Hautkr.*; **66**: 968–70.

CHAPTER TWELVE

OCCUPATIONAL SKIN INFECTIONS

John T Lear and John SC English

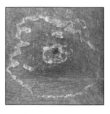

Staphylococcal infections are usually secondary to occupational lacerations and abrasions.

Secondary syphilis.

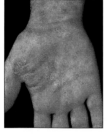

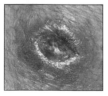

Cutaneous Leishmaniasis in a soldier who had been training in the jungle.

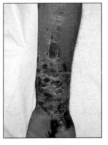

Cutaneous anthrax.

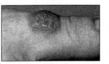

Fishtank granuloma from *Mycobacterium marinum*.

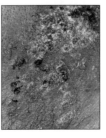

Inflammatory cattle ringworm in a dairy farmer.

INTRODUCTION

Many occupations can be associated with a risk of infection particularly when conditions favour disease transmission. Bacteria can affect individuals exposed, in the course of their work, to infected humans, animals or their products. Similarly, viruses can be transmitted in this way but may also infect laboratory personnel processing infected products. Parasites can affect those with predominantly outdoor occupations and fungal disease can be acquired in tropical and subtropical climates, especially in agricultural workers. Family members of people with such occupations are also at risk. Establishing an occupational cause for a particular infection can be a difficult task. History, the nature of the occupation and microbiological investigations can all help. This chapter will review the known causes of occupational skin infections concentrating on the commoner conditions encountered in clinical practice.

BACTERIAL INFECTIONS

Occupational bacterial infections are listed in *Table 36*.

Staphylococci and *Streptococci*

Secondary infection from lacerations, burns, puncture wounds and abrasions are the most common staphylococcal or streptococcal infections. Construction and farm workers are at risk of folliculitis and boils (**311**). Boners, animal killers and meat packers can develop pustular and inflamed lesions with the infected meat acting as a vehicle of transmission. Staphylococcal ecthyma in a fish seller has been reported. It seems likely that these often trivial superficial infections are widely under-reported. Also, contaminated cutting oils may carry infection and put individuals at risk in their workplace.

Anthrax

Bacillus anthracis can affect cattle, sheep, goats, buffaloes and camels; they are infected by eating grass on contaminated soil. The organism can remain viable in the dead animal for long periods particularly in the skin, bowel, fleece and hair leading to a considerable occupational hazard. Infection is usually cutaneous, particularly on the exposed sites with, classically, a black pustule, later lymphangitis and a febrile illness (**312**). Vigorous safeguards have been used to minimise infection but its risk is still marked where these procedures are not followed.

Wool sorters were classically affected with the inhalation of spores leading to the development of pulmonary anthrax (wool sorter's disease). Anyone handling hair, meat or hides (e.g. dock workers, butchers and agricultural workers) can also be affected. The treatment of choice is penicillin and tetracycline. Incision and drainage should be avoided as this procedure can lead to systemic dissemination. Prevention can be achieved by anti-anthrax vaccination of susceptible animals, elimination of soil pollution and decontamination of hides. These measures have been used successfully in the USA since the 1930s.

Table 36. Occupational bacterial infections.

Bacterium	Occupations at special risk
Staphylococcus aureus	Explorers; butchers; fish sellers
Streptococci	Farm workers; butchers; fish sellers
Bacillus anthracis	Brick workers; dockers; wool sorters; butchers; hide and hair workers
Brucella abortis/suis/melitensis	Abattoir workers; veterinarians; meat packers
Erysipelothrix rhusiopathiae	Vets; fishermen; butchers; poultry dressers
Mycobacterium tuberculosis	Surgeons; vets; farmers; butchers
Mycobacterium marinum	Fishermen; fish tank cleaners
Salmonella dublin	Vets
Yersinia pseudotuberculosis/enterocolitica	Farmers; bird/pigeon handlers
Francisella tularensis	Farmers; vets; butchers; foresters
Treponema pallidum	Prostitutes; glassblowers; laboratory and medical personnel
Corynebacteria	Soldiers
Leptospira icterohaemorrhagicae/canicola	Sewer workers
Relapsing fever	Animal handlers/zoo attendants

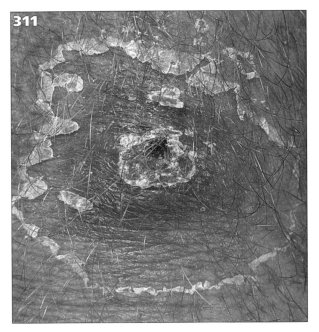

311 Staphylococcal furuncle.

312 Cutaneous anthrax: multiple black pustules.

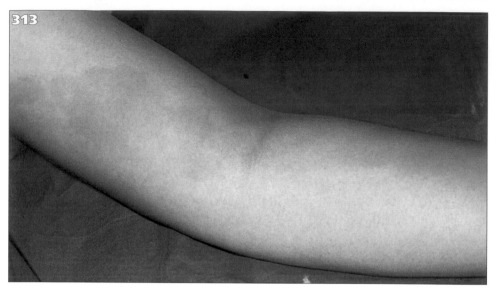

313 Brucellosis: urticarial wheal.

Brucellosis

This may be seen in vets, abattoir workers, meat packers and laboratory technicians. It is an acute illness with fever and prostration, possibly followed by a chronic form with splenic abscesses, renal disease and bladder involvement. Three types exist: *Brucella suis*, found in pigs; *Brucella abortus*, found in cattle; and *Brucella melitensis*, found in sheep and goats. Infection is through contact with contaminated animals or by ingesting infected milk and cheese. Non-specific skin manifestations are seen, ranging from a maculopapular eruption to petechiae to chronic ulcers. A contact-type urticaria may be seen (313) with subsequent vesico-pustule formation which is thought to represent a hypersensitivity reaction to the bacterial antigen.

Preventative measures include the elimination of infected animals and the vaccination of healthy ones. Human vaccination with a live vaccine can be effective. Treatment with oxytetracycline 500 mg qds for 3 weeks is usually adequate. The chronic form is more difficult to eradicate.

Erysipeloid (fish-handler's disease)

The causative organism, *Erysipelothrix rhusiopathiae*, infests fish, shellfish and poultry. Breaks in the skin provide a portal of entry although it can penetrate intact skin. At-risk occupations include fishermen, butchers and poultry dressers. Infection is seen on the hands with a painful, purplish papule and a spreading, dusky erythema with lymphadenitis. Septicaemia may occur. Prevention can be achieved by eliminating decaying nitrogenous material and strict factory hygiene. Penicillin is the treatment of choice.

Fishtank granuloma

This is caused by *Mycobacterium marinum* and most patients acquire it from infected fish or aquariums. Gulf fishermen and fishtank cleaners are at greatest risk. Granulomatous papules and nodules (**314**) which can ulcerate are seen with a characteristic spread along local lymphatics. Tetracycline is the treatment of choice.

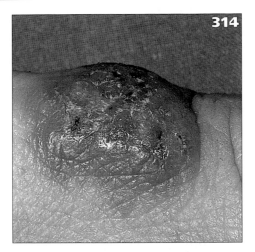

314 Fishtank granuloma: nodule on the thumb of a tropical fishtank cleaner.

Syphilis

Non-venereal syphilis was traditionally a hazard for glassblowers who shared mouthpieces but it may also affect medical personnel and laboratory technicians. Any occupation facilitating sexual intercourse with numerous partners is associated with an increased risk of venereal syphilis and its sequelae (**315**).

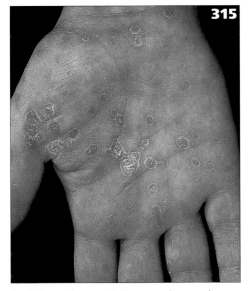

315 Secondary syphilis: maculo-papular rash on the palm.

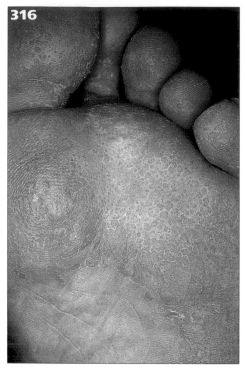

316 Pitted keratolysis: circular erosions on the foot.

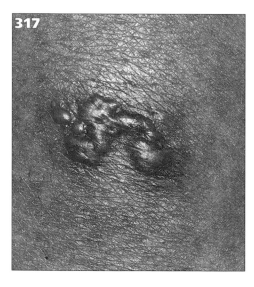

317 *Herpes simplex*: coalescent vesicles.

Pitted keratolysis

This condition is facilitated by excessive sweating and occlusion of the feet. Occupationally it is seen in those wearing boots for long periods of time, for example soldiers, miners and labourers. It can be quite troublesome forcing some to leave their jobs. Circular erosions on the feet is the typical clinical picture (316); hyperhidrosis is usually associated. Treatment of the hyperhidrosis improves the condition and sodium fusidate cream can help. Other topical antibiotics and imidazoles have been used.

VIRAL INFECTIONS

Occupational viral infections are listed in *Table 37*.

Herpes simplex

Herpes simplex, either type 1 or 2, is a well-recognised cause of hand infections. Professions at increased risk include health personnel and dentists exposed to oral or respiratory tract secretions. A herpetic whitlow can be seen with localised swelling and erythema and local lymphadenopathy. Coalescent vesicles may occur later (317).

Table 37. Occupational viral infections.

Virus	Occupations at special risk
Herpes simplex	Medical/dental personnel
Poxviruses (including paravaccinia type)	Vets; sheep herders; farmers; animal shearers; butchers
Human papilloma	Butchers; other meat handlers
Paravaccinia	Cow milkers; vets
HIV	Laboratory and medical personnel
Cow pox	Cattle workers

Orf (*Ecthyma contagiosum*)

This is caused by a *paravaccinia* sub-group of poxviruses and is endemic in sheep and goats causing pustular stomatitis in the new-born animals. Transmission to humans is by direct contact usually via a break in the skin. A macule appears 4 days after inoculation which evolves into a papule with a red centre and a surrounding white ring. A granulomatous lesion followed by ulceration with healing without scarring completes the natural history of the lesion (318, 319). Lesions may be multiple. At greatest risk are sheep herders, vets and farmers.

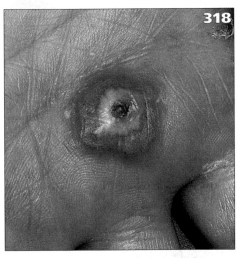

318 Orf: papule with red centre and surrounding white ring.

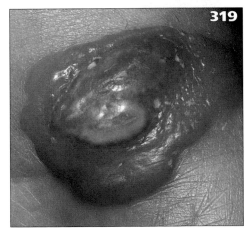

319 Orf: granulomatous lesion.

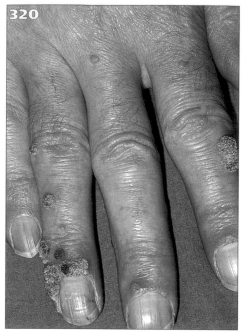

320 Viral warts.

Human papilloma virus

Butchers and other meat handlers may acquire viral warts in the course of their work probably due to a combination of trauma, low working temperatures and humidity (320). HPV 7 is isolated more commonly in these warts than those acquired non-occupationally.

Milker's nodules

This *paravaccinia* virus causes nodules on the hands and forearms which resemble orf (321, 322). It is transmitted via infected cows and is seen in dairy farmers, vets and in newly employed farm workers who have not developed immunity. Hand milking is high risk for exposure to the virus. Regional lymphadenopathy may be present. Resolution is spontaneous and prevention via use of rubber gloves, isolation of infected cows and hygienic milking procedures is effective. Wild rodents have been reported to transmit cow pox in Poland.

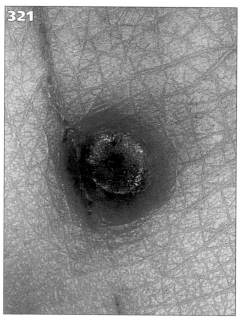

321 Milker's nodules: nodule resembling orf on the hand of a dairy farmer.

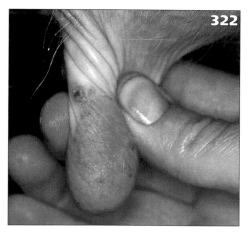

322 Milker's nodules: papules on the udder of an infected cow.

FUNGAL AND YEAST INFECTIONS

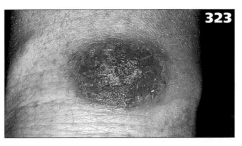

323 Tinea: scaly lesion on the forearm.

Occupational fungal and yeast infections are listed in *Table 38*.

Dermatophytes

Occupations at risk include those in contact with animals or soil products and those working in humid, traumatising and occlusive circumstances. An occupational relationship is established by isolating the same dermatophyte from the worker and the animals in their care. Scaly lesions on the hands or inflammatory lesions are found in infected humans (**323, 324**). *Trichophyton verrucosum* is mostly associated with cattle infection and humans may be affected directly or via contamination from barns, fences and straw. The fungus is viable for 1 year in the environment. Inflammatory lesions can be seen. *T. mentagrophytes* can be transmitted by cattle and domestic animals including cats and dogs. It can affect all areas but is a common cause of tinea

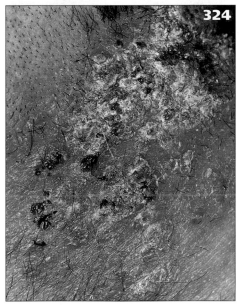

324 Tinea: inflammatory patch with hair loss.

Table 38. Occupational fungal and yeast infections.

Fungus	Occupations at special risk
Dermatophytes	Farm workers; zoo attendants; explorers; laboratory technicians; agricultural workers; miners
Candida albicans	Caterers; cleaners; bartenders; cutting oil machinists; dishwashers
Malassezia furfur	Explorers; tropical climate workers
Sporothrix schenckii	Nursery/agricultural/forestry workers; miners
Blastomyces dermatitidis	Laboratory workers
Mycetoma	Agricultural workers
Chromomycosis	Agricultural workers
Coccidiodes immitis	Migrant workers; military personnel; bulldozer operators

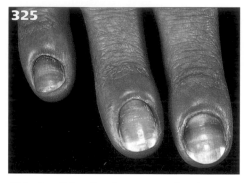

325 Candida: discoloration and nail dystrophy with paronychia.

pedis. Barn workers are at risk of this infection. *T. rubrum* is seen in sportsmen and miners. *Microsporum nanum* can affect pig workers and present as scaly erythematous patches indistinguishable clinically from other fungal infections. Pet shop workers and vets can contract *M. canis* infections from small animals. *M. gypseum* is found in soil containing clay and can affect agricultural workers. Sharing shower facilities can also increase fungus transmission. Oral antifungal agents are usually necessary to clear these infections.

Candida infections

This constitutes the most common fungal occupationally acquired infection. The hands and fingernails are usually affected with intertrigo, desquamation and nail dystrophy (325). Paronychia can be seen. At-risk occupations include dishwashing, laundering, food handling and exposure to cutting oils (via irritancy and degreasing effects on the skin).

RICKETTSIAL INFECTIONS

Most of these infections are transmitted by blood-sucking insects and mites; farmers, trappers, rangers, hunters, surveyors and guides are at risk (*Table 39*, 326). Skin manifestations include maculo-papular eruptions which can become haemorrhagic with associated fever.

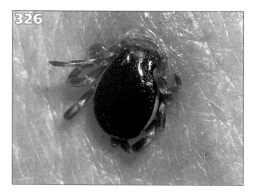

326 Blood-sucking insect engorging itself.

Table 39. Occupational rickettsial infections.

Type	Occupations at special risk
Tick typhus	–
Scrub typhus	Explorers; farmers
Murine typhus	Abattoir workers; guides; trappers
Epidemic typhus	Surveyors; sodiers; foresters
Rocky Mountain spotted fever	–

PARASITIC INFECTIONS

Occupational parasitic infections are listed in *Table 40*.

Scabies

This is caused by the organism *Sarcoptes scabiei*. Any occupation dealing with large numbers of people involving close or sexual contact is at risk of scabies, for example medical personnel and prostitutes. Scabies can also be contracted by close contact with dogs – it can be seen in dog handlers. The animal in suspected cases should be examined for para-sites. In people, characteristic burrows are seen classically between the finger web spaces (**327**) and a generalised papular rash can occur. Diagnosis can be difficult but papules on the genitalia are a helpful diagnostic sign. Burrows should be scraped to enable microscopic visualisation of the mite to confirm diagnosis.

Protozoa

Mucocutaneous Leishmaniasis is transmitted via small flies endemic in warm climates. Workers in tropical forests are

Table 40. Occupational parasitic infections.	
Parasite	**Occupations at special risk**
Sarcoptes scabiei	Medical personnel; salesmen; soldiers
Leishmania tropica	Tropical forest workers; soldiers
Ancylostoma braziliense/duodenale	Beach workers; sewer workers; ditch diggers
Insecta	Outdoor occupations
Borrelia burgdorferi	Outdoor workers; loggers
Schistosoma	Rice planters; canal workers
Echinococci	Shepherds; farmers
Toxocara	Dog breeders
Cercariae	Divers; lifeguards; pond workers

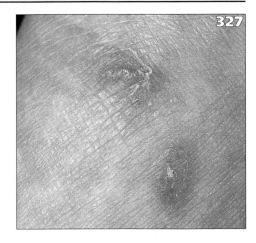

327 Scabies: burrows on the palm.

179

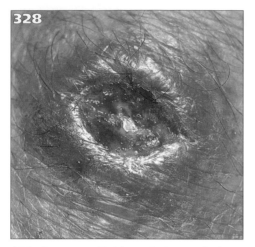

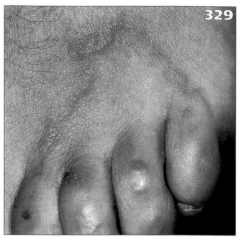

328 Cutaneous Leishmaniasis: punched out ulcer.

329 Larva migrans: red, raised line on the foot.

at increased risk of this condition which presents as an ulcer but can later become scarring and nodular (328).

Helminths

Larva migrans (creeping eruption)

This is caused by a variety of nematodes, most commonly by *Ancylostoma braziliense* in the USA. The faeces of cattle and dogs contain the larvae and transmission to humans occurs when contact is made with contaminated soil, particularly on sandy beaches where the faeces are not readily visible. A slightly red, raised line is seen, usually on the feet (329). This is due to larval movement which can be up to 1 cm a day. Treatment is with 10% topical thiobendazole.

Cercarial dermatitis (swimmer's itch)

This is caused by the cercariae of a schistosome producing a highly pruritic eruption with urticaria and papules. It lasts

for a week or two and can become secondarily infected. It is classically seen in a bathing costume distribution as the cercariae get trapped in the costume and only sting when they cannot move away from the body. Divers, lifeguards, dock workers and pond workers have all been reported in association with this condition. Treatment is symptomatic. Prevention may be achieved by treating infected water with copper sulphate.

Arthropods

Outdoor occupations such as farming are at increased risk of various insect, spider and beetle bites and their sequelae. Reactions to toxins or allergenic proteins account for the clinical manifestations. Lyme disease is caused by the organism *Borrelia burgdorferi* and is transmitted by the Ixodes tick. Outdoor workers are at increased risk. A characteristic rash is seen (erythema chronicum migrans). This is due to the local spread of the spirochete usually in a ring formation which gradually enlarges. The erythema can be slight or intense. A zone of clearing may be seen behind the advancing ring. Serology is helpful in diagnosis although this may be negative in the first few weeks. Later arthralgia, arthritis, neurological and cardiac abnormalities may be seen. Early treatment with a three week course of penicillin (amoxycillin 500–1000 mg three times daily) can prevent serious later sequelae.

BIBLIOGRAPHY

Adams, RM (1990), *Occupational Skin Disease*, W.B. Saunders Co., Philadelphia.

Champion, RH, Burton, JL and Ebling, FJG (1992), *Textbook of Dermatology*, Blackwell Scientific Publications, Oxford.

Weatherall, DJ, Ledingham, JGG and Warrel, DA (1996), *Oxford Textbook of Medicine*, OUP, Oxford.

INDEX

A

Acanthosis, 20
Acids, as irritants, 12, 22, 67
Acne (occupational), 121–134
  coal tar, 130, 131
  oil acne, 122–124
  treatment, 124
  tropical, 134
Acne aestivalis (mallorca acne), 132
Acne cosmetica, 132
Acne mechanica, 71, 132–133
Acne venenata, 122
Acne vulgaris, chloracne comparison, 130
Acrodermatitis perstans, 95
Acropustulosis, 95
Acrosclerosis, 161
Acrylates, fingertip dermatitis, 46
Acrylic monomers, 68, 76, 85, 89, 93
Actinic dermatitis photosensitivity, chronic, 60, 116
Actinic reticuloid syndrome, 48, 49
  photosensitivity dermatitis (PD/AR), 60, 61
Acute irritant reactions, 12–13
Age, irritant contact dermatitis, 21
Alkalis, as irritants, 12, 22
Alkyl phenols, 154
Allergens
  airborne, 36, 38, 50
  avoidance, 51
  patch tests, 8, 33–34
  plants, 113
Allergic contact dermatitis, 31–52
  at-risk occupations, 34, 35
  causes, and appearances due to, 38–50
    acrylates, 46
    acrylic monomers, 68, 76, 85, 89, 93
    chromate, 38, 39, 64
    cobalt, 40
    colophony, 44–45, 68
    epoxy/epoxy resins, 46–47, 65, 66
    formaldehyde/formaldehyde resins, 44, 69
    fragrances, 47
    miscellaneous, 50–51, 70, 71, 73, 74, 76, 87, 93, 94, 95, 101
    nickel, 40–42, 74, 76, 88
    plants, 48–49, 88, 92, 113–119

Allergic contact dermatitis (*cont.*)
  causes, and appearances due to (*cont.*)
    rubber/rubber gloves, 36, 43, 70, 71, 86
    wood, 118–119
  clinical features, 34–38, 68–74
  differential diagnosis, 85, 86, 87–88, 101
  elicitation, 32–34
  fingertip, 36, 37, 45, 46, 50, 93–94
  hairdressers, 50, 73, 83, 93, 94, 96
  investigations, 8, 33
  irritant contact dermatitis *vs*, 15, 87–88
  management, 51–52
  pompholyx-like, 100
  secondary infection, 96–97
  sensitisation, 32
Allergic contact urticaria, 50
Alstroemeria, 48, 88, 92, 114
American Rheumatism Association, 166
Amiodarone, phototoxicity, 56
Ancylostoma braziliense, 180
'Angry back', 33
Anthrax, 170, 171
Antibiotics, allergic contact dermatitis, 50
Antigens, 32, 34
Aprons, contact dermatitis prevention, 28
Argyria, 156–157
Arsenic, 138–140
Arthropod infestations, 180–181
Asteatotic eczema, 95
Atopic dermatitis, 21, 83, 89
  hand, 89
Atopy, 89

B

Bacillus anthracis, 170
Bacterial infections, 170–174
Bakers, 50, 51
Barrier creams, 9, 28, 52
Basal cell carcinoma, 139, 140, 141, 143
Beauticians, 76
Benzanthrone, 59
Benzo(a)pyrene, 137
Benzocaine-containing creams, 77
Biocides, 44, 73, 74
Boils, 170
Boots, *see* Footwear
Borage, 106
Borrelia burgdorferi, 180

Bowens disease, 144
Brassica oleracea, 108, 109
Brucellosis, 172
Bulbs, fingertip dermatitis, 92, 106, 107, 114
Bullous allergic contact dermatitis, 113
Bullous phototoxic reaction, 110
Burns, 12–13
  cement, 24
  chemical, 12, 77
  chromic acid, 23
  hydrofluoric acid, 23

C

Cactus species, 105
'California Glory', 105
Candida infections, 178
Car mechanics, 86
Car tyres, 70, 71
Celery, 58, 112
Cell-mediated immunity, 32–34
Cement
  burns, 24
  contact dermatitis, 24, 64
  as irritant, 24
Ceramides, 20
Cercarial dermatitis (swimmer's itch), 180
Chapping, 86
Chefs
  allergic contact dermatitis, 34, 35, 36, 37, 72, 99
  irritant contact dermatitis, 6, 26
  post-occupational dermatitis, 98
Cheilitis, allergic, 117
Chemical burns, 12, 77
Chemicals
  acute irritant reactions/burns, 12
  occupational vitiligo, 149–151
Chicory, 106, 107
Chimney sweeps, 136–137
Chloracne, 122, 123, 124–131
  acne vulgaris *vs*, 130
  clinical features, 126, 127–129
  differential diagnosis, 130, 131
  histology, 126
  non-occupational, 124
  retroauricular, 126, 128
  treatment and prevention, 131
Chloracnegens, 124, 125, 126
Chlorobenzene chloracne, 122, 127, 128, 129, 130
Chlorpromazine, 62
Chromate dermatitis, 38, 39, 64

'Chrome cripple', 5
Chrome ulcer, 23
Chromic acid, 22
  burns, 23
Chrysanthemum, allergy, 88,
  114–115
Clay, 74, 78
Cleaners, dermatitis in, 15, 78,
  83
Coal tar acne, 130, 131
Coal tattoo, 80
Cobalt allergy, 40
Coins, nickel allergy and, 42
Cold sores, 55
Cold urticaria, 78
Colophony, 44–45, 68,
  116–117
Comedones, chloracne, 126,
  127
Compositae plants, 38, 48, 49,
  116
Connective tissue disorders,
  occupational, 159–168
Contact allergy, multiple, to
  plants, 60, 61
Contact dermatitis, occupation-
  al, 4, 64–77
  aetiology, 6
  age groups, 4
  allergic, see Allergic contact
    dermatitis
  costs, 3
  frequency/prevalence, 2, 3
  investigations, 8
  irritant, see Irritant contact
    dermatitis
  patterns, 7
  prevention, 9–10
  prognosis, 5
Contact urticaria, 34
Contractures, 164
Costs, occupational contact dermatitis, 3
Cow parsley, 112
Creeping eruption (larva
  migrans), 180
p-Cresol, 149, 150
Cumulative insult dermatitis, see
  Irritant contact dermatitis
Cutis rhomboidalis nuchae, 55
Cutting fluids, as irritants, 26,
  27
Cutting oils, 65, 122, 138
Cyanide, inorganic, 13, 22
1,2-Cyclohexane dicarboxylic
  acid, bis (oxyrinylmethyl)
  ester, 65, 66
Cysts, straw-coloured, 126, 127,
  128

D
Dairy farmers, viral infections,
  176
'Damping down', dust, 119
Dandelion dermatitis, 116
Delayed pressure urticaria, 78

Delayed-type (type 4) hypersen-
  sitivity, 32–34, 72, 87
Dental assistants/technicians,
  36, 46, 163
Dentists, 68
Depigmentation, 148–155
  see also Leukoderma
Dermatitis, 3, 64–77
  acute weeping, 28
  secondarily infected, 96–97
  see also Contact dermatitis;
    specific types of dermatitis
Dermatomyositis, 168
Dermatophyte infections, 177
Detergents, as irritant, 22, 67
Diallyl sulphide, 37
Dichromates, 5, 38, 39
Dictamnus albus, 111
Dieffenbachia picta, 108
Dimethylglyoxime test, 40, 41
Dimethyl thiourea, 100
Dioxins, 126
Discoid eczema, 26, 27, 100
Dog handlers, 179
Drugs, phototoxic, 57
Dyes, dermatitis, 69
Dyshidrosis lamellosa sicca, 94

E
Ecthyma, staphylococcal, 170
Ecthyma contagiosum, 175
Eczema, 82–102
  discoid, 26, 27, 100
  see also Dermatitis; Hand
Eczema craquelé, 95
'Eczema nails', 36, 38
Eczematous reaction, 33, 68
Elastotic changes, 55
Electronics industry, 40, 41, 42
Emollients, 9, 28
'Endogenous' eczema, 97
EPI-DERM, 3
Epoxy resins, allergic contact
  dermatitis, 46–47, 65, 66
Erosions, skin, 12, 13, 174
Erysipeloid (fish-handler's dis-
  ease), 172
Erysipelothrix rhusiopathiae,
  172
Erythema chronicum migrans,
  180
Ethylenediamine, 101
Euphorbia species, 107

F
Face
  allergic contact dermatitis, 38,
    47, 50, 68, 116, 117
  pigmentation changes, 151,
    157
Farmers, 50, 55, 140, 180
Feet, pitted keratolysis, 174
Fibreglass, 24, 25
Fibroblasts, 167
Ficus carica, 111
'Fiddler's neck', 71, 133

Fingers
  allergic contact dermatitis, 35,
    36, 40, 88
  contractures, 164
Fingertip dermatitis, 84
  allergic contact dermatitis, 36,
    37, 45, 46, 50, 93–94
  atopic, 89
  plants causing, 92, 106, 107,
    114
Fingertip psoriasis, 92, 93
Finger web dermatitis, 7, 16, 85,
  116
Fish, allergy, 6, 72
Fish-handler's disease
  (erysipeloid), 172
Fishtank granuloma, 173
Fissures, hands, 85, 86
Florists, allergic contact dermatitis, 48, 88, 92, 114–115
Folliculitis, 170
  oil, 18, 123, 130
Food handlers
  allergic contact dermatitis, 34,
    35, 36, 37
  immediate contact dermatitis,
    98, 99
  irritant contact dermatitis, 72
  urticaria, 108
  see also Chefs
Foods, as irritants, 26
  allergic contact urticaria, 50
Footwear
  allergic contact dermatitis and,
    40, 42, 71
  irritant contact dermatitis pre-
    vention, 28
Formaldehyde, allergic contact
  dermatitis, 44, 69
Fragrances, allergic contact dermatitis, 47
Frictional trauma, 71, 73, 79,
  84
Frost-bite, 79
Fungal infections, 82, 92,
  177–178
Furniture industry, 118–119
Furuncle, staphylococcal, 171

G
Gardeners, 56, 60, 61, 107,
  112, 116
  facial dermatitis, 117
Garlic, 36, 37, 106
Gases, as irritants, 12
Gender, irritant contact dermatitis, 21
Gloves, 9, 28
  allergic contact dermatitis, 34,
    36, 43, 51–52, 71
  contamination, 51–52
  latex, 34, 36, 44
  prevention of contact dermati-
    tis, 9, 28
  rubber, depigmentation due
    to, 148–149

Gloves (*cont.*)
rubber additives, 43, 44
thiuram allergy, 86
types/materials, 10
Glues, locking, 68, 76
Glyceryl monothioglycolate, 73, 83, 93
Glycosylceramides, 20
Gold cyanide, 13, 22
Gut-eczema, 99

H
Hairdressers, 50, 73, 83
allergic contact dermatitis, 50, 73, 83, 93, 94, 96
cumulative irritant contact dermatitis, 85
sub-acute allergic contact dermatitis, 87
Halogen acne, *see* Chloracne
Hand, 81–102
acropustulosis, 95
allergic contact dermatitis, 35, 48, 87–88
differential diagnosis, 85, 87–88
secondary infection, 96, 97
see also Allergic contact dermatitis
asteatotic eczema, 95
atopic dermatitis, 89
dermatitis prevalence, 2
discoid eczema, 100
eczema, differential diagnosis, 81–102
fissures and cracks, 85, 86
frictional dermatitis, 73, 84
fungus infection, 83, 92
hyperkeratotic dermatitis, 90, 91
immediate contact reaction, 98–99
irritant contact dermatitis, acute, 67
clinical features, 64, 65, 67, 72, 73, 75
cumulative insult, 15, 20, 25, 27, 64, 65, 85–87
differential diagnosis, 85–87
water/detergents/soap, 15, 22, 67, 84
keratolysis exfoliativa, 94
mechanical trauma, 73, 84, 85
neurodermatitis circumscripta, 101
persistent palmar pustulosis, 96
phototoxic/photoallergic reactions, 101
pompholyx, 99–100
post-occupational eczema, 97–98
post-traumatic eczema, 73, 97
protein contact dermatitis, 34, 35
psoriasis, 90, 91, 92
secondarily infected dermatitis, 96–97

Hand (*cont.*)
trauma, 73
see also Allergic contact dermatitis; Fingers; Irritant contact dermatitis
Haptens, 32
Hardwoods, 118, 119
Health education, 29
Helminth infections, 180
Henna, 108
Herpes simplex virus infections, 174, 175
Human papilloma virus, 176
Hutchinson's melanotic freckle, 144
Hydrofluoric acid, 22, 23
Hydroquinone, 148, 149, 150, 152, 153
Hygiene, personal, 9, 51
Hyperhidrosis, 174
Hyperkeratosis, 20
follicular, 122, 126
oil, 141
sub-ungual, 93
Hyperkeratotic dermatitis, 90, 91
Hyperpigmentation, 110
chloracne, 126, 129
coal tar acne, 131
Hypersensitivity
delayed-type (type 4), 32–34, 72, 89
immediate-type, 34, 72, 98, 108
Hypopigmentation, 148–155
post-inflammatory, 148
systemic sclerosis, 165
see also Leukoderma

I
Immediate contact reactions, 98–99
Immediate-type hypersensitivity, 34, 72, 98, 108
Immunoglobulin E (IgE), 34
Infections, *see* Skin infections
Inflammatory mediators, 19
Insecticides, 138
Investigations, 8
see also Patch tests
Ionising radiation, skin cancer, 138, 139
IPPD (4-isopropylamino-diphenylamine), 43
Iroko dermatitis, 119
Irritant contact dermatitis, 11–29
acute, 14, 17, 19, 67
after pre-existing dermatitis, 21
allergic contact dermatitis *vs*, 15, 87–88
at-risk occupations, 9, 17, 22
chronic (cumulative insult), 15, 17, 19, 27, 85–87, 89
clinical features, 12, 14–17, 64–65, 67, 73, 75, 83

Irritant contact dermatitis (*cont.*)
definition, 12
diagnosis, 15, 21, 84–85
differential diagnosis, 84–86
epidemiology, 12
food handlers, 72
hands, *see* Hand
histology, 19, 20
irritants, 14, 17, 22–27, 65
mechanism, 19–20
plants and wood exposure, 105–108
predisposing risk factors, 21
secondary infection, 97
sites, 14, 16, 85
treatment and prevention, 28–29
Irritant skin reactions, classification, 12
Irritants, skin, 12, 17, 22–27, 65
weak, 14
Isopropyl phenyl-*p*-phenylenediamine (IPPD), 70, 71, 94
Itching, 87

K
Kathon CG, 73, 74
Keratolysis, pitted, 174
Keratolysis exfoliativa, 94
Koebnerisation, 79

L
Lamellar desquamation, 94
Lancashire Mule Spinners, 137
Langerhan's cells, 32
Larva migrans (creeping eruption), 180
Latex
gloves, 34, 36, 44
prick test, 44
urticaria, 44
see also Rubber
Leather tanning, 38, 39, 148
Leishmaniasis, mucocutaneous, 179, 180
Lentigo maligna melanoma, 144, 145
Leukoderma (vitiligo), occupational, 148–155
at-risk occupations, 154
chemicals causing, 149–151
clinical features, 151–154
diagnosis, 154
management, 154
mechanism/pathogenesis, 154–155
Leyland cypress, 117
Lichenified eczema, 101
Lichen planus, 79, 102
Light, artificial, 56
occupational disorders associated, 53–62
Lithographers, 75
Loctite™, 68, 76
Lupus erythematosus, 167
Lyme disease, 180

M

McDonald's acne, 122
Machine tool industry, 65, 122, 138
Mallorca acne (acne aestivalis), 132
Meat handlers, 176
Meat packers, 170, 172
Mechanical trauma, 84, 85
  dermatitis, 73, 84, 85, 101
  irritant reactions to plants, 105–106
  see also Frictional trauma
Melanocytes, depigmentation mechanism, 154, 155
Melanoma, malignant, 140, 141, 145
  management, 146
  nodular, 144, 145
  superficial spreading, 144, 145
Mercaptobenzothiazole, 43
Metalworkers, 26
Methyldibromoglutaronitril, 95
Microsporum species, 178
Miliaria, 18
Milker's nodules, 176
Mineral oil, skin cancer, 137–138
Miners, 80
Monkfish, allergy, 6
Monobenzylether of hydro-quinone, 148, 149, 150
Monomethylether of hydro-quinone, 150
Mononuclear cell infiltration, 19
Morphoea, 167
Mycobacterium marinum, 173

N

Nail
  argyria, 157
  cumulative irritant contact dermatitis, 86
  dystrophy, 36, 38
Nailfold infarcts, 164
Nail technicians, 76, 89
Narcissus pseudonarcissus, 106
Neurodermatitis circumscripta, 101
Nickel, 40–42
  allergy (contact dermatitis), 40–42, 74, 76, 88
  cumulative irritant contact dermatitis, 88
  patch tests, 33
  spot test, 40, 41
Nitrogen mustard gas burns, 13
Nodules, milker's, 176
Non-eczematous skin reactions, 18
Nummular eczema, 100

O

Occupations, at-risk
  bacterial infections, 170, 172
  dermatitis/urticaria, 3

Occupations, at-risk (cont.)
  fungal infections, 177, 178
  irritant contact dermatitis, 9, 17, 22
  parasitic infections, 179
  phototoxic reactions due to plants, 111
  pigmentation changes, 154, 158
  plants and wood exposure, 104
  rickettsial infections, 178
  scleroderma, 163
  skin cancer, 136
  ultraviolet exposure, 54
  viral infections, 175
  vitiligo (leukoderma), 154
Oil(s)
  cooking, 124
  coolant, 65
  cutting, 65, 122, 138
  mineral, skin cancer, 137–138
  skin cancer and, 138
  synthetic water-soluble, 26, 27
Oil acne, 122–124
Oil boils, 122
Oil folliculitis, 18, 123, 130
Onycholysis, 76, 79
Orf (ecthyma contagiosum), 175
Organic salts, as irritants, 12

P

Palmar pustulosis, persistent, 96
Parasitic infections, 179–181
Parsley, 106, 113
Parsnips, 109, 112
Patch tests, 8, 15, 33, 87
  allergens used, 8, 33–34
  hand eczema, 82
  hardwoods, 118
  positive and false-positive, 33
  principle/pitfalls, 33
Persistent light reaction, 75
Persistent occupational dermatitis, 64, 97–98
Persistent palmar pustulosis, 96
Peruvian Lily, see Alstroemeria
Pesticides, 138
Phenol formaldehyde resin, 69
Phenols, occupational vitiligo, 149, 150, 154
p-Phenylene-diamine, 70, 71, 94
Photoallergy, 60, 62, 75, 101
Photocontact reactions, 60
Photodermatoses, idiopathic, 60–62
Photosensitisers, 56, 57, 75
Photosensitivity
  dermatitis/actinic reticuloid syndrome (PD/AR), 60, 61
Phototoxicity, 56–59
  agents causing, 56, 57
Phototoxic reactions, 101
  plants, 58, 59, 101, 109–112
  prevention, 113
Phytophotodermatitis, 58, 59, 101, 109–112

Pigmentary changes, occupational, 147–158
Pigmentation, colours and causes, 158
Pitch, skin cancer, 137
Pitch acne, 130, 131
Pityriasis lichenoides, 112
Plants, occupational dermatitis, 103–119
  allergens, 113
  allergic contact dermatitis, 48, 49, 88, 92, 113–119
  fingertip dermatitis, 114
  irritant reactions, 105–108
  multiple contact allergy, 60, 61
  phototoxic reactions, 58, 59, 101, 109–112
  prevention, 113
  sap, irritant, 106
  urticaria, 108–109
  see also specific plants
Poisoning, systemic, 122, 124
Poison ivy (Rhus), 113
Polychlorinated biphenyls (PCBs), 124
Polycyclic hydrocarbons, 136–138
Polymorphic light reaction, 60–61
Pompholyx, 99–100
Post-exogenous eczema, 97
Post-occupational eczema, 97–98
Post-traumatic eczema, 97
Potassium dichromate, 5
Potatoes, protein contact dermatitis, 35, 108
Pottery industry, 4, 74, 75
Poxviruses, 175
Prechloracne lesions, 126
Pre-employment examination/screening, 9, 28
Prickly pear, 105
Prick testing, 108
Primula dermatitis, 48, 49, 116
Printers, 85, 93, 97
Protein contact dermatitis, 34, 35, 50, 51, 108
Protozoan infections, 179–180
Pruriginous eruptions, 24, 26
Psoralen phytophotodermatitis, 58
Psoralens, 57, 109, 110, 112
Psoriasis, 4, 85, 91
  fingertip, 92, 93
  hands, 85, 90, 91
  palmar, 90, 91
Pustules, 96
  black (anthrax), 170, 171

Q

Quarternium 15, 7
Quartz, 162, 163, 166
  lupus erythematosus, 168
Quartz-induced scleroderma, 162–167

185

Quartz-induced scleroderma (*cont.*)
clinical/pathological features, 163–165
pathogenesis, 166–167
Quinine, photoleucomelanoderma, 57

R
Race, irritant contact dermatitis, 21
Radiograph envelopes, 45
Radiotherapy, 138
Rat-bite necrosis, 164
Raynaud's phenomenon, 167, 168
Rhus, 113
Rice cooking oil, 124
Rickettsial infections, 178
Rubber
accelerator/additives, 43, 44, 70, 71
allergic contact dermatitis, 36, 43, 70, 71, 86
see also Gloves; Latex
Rubber tree, 108
Rue, 111, 113

S
Sabra dermatitis, 105
Sarcoptes scabiei, 179
Scabies, 179
Schistosomiasis, 180
Scleroderma, 160, 162, 163
at-risk occupations, 163
clinical features, 163–165
diagnostic criteria, 166
localised (morphoea), 167
see also Quartz-induced scleroderma
Scleroderma-like disease, 160–161
Scrotal squamous carcinoma, 136, 137
Sensitisation, 32
Sesquiterpene lactones, 48, 49
Shale oil, 137
Silicon dioxide (quartz), 162, 163, 166
Silicone breast implants,163
Silicosis, 168
pulmonary, 162
Silver, argyria, 156–157
Skin cancer, occupational, 135–146
arsenic causing, 138–140
at-risk occupations, 136
causative agents, 136
diagnosis, 141–145
ionising radiation, 138, 139
management, 146
polycyclic hydrocarbons, 136–137, 138
ultraviolet light, 140–141
Skin cleansers, 9, 28

Skin infections, occupational, 169–182
bacterial, 170–174
fungal, 82, 92, 177–178
parasitic, 179–181
rickettsial, 178
secondary, 28, 96–97
viral, 174–176
Slaughterhouse workers, 79, 99
Smoking, 140, 144
Soaps, as irritant, 22
Sodium lauryl sulphate, 21
Solar elastosis, 55
Solar keratoses, 142
Solar urticaria, 61
Solderers, 14, 25
Solder fumes, 68
Soldering fluxes, as irritants, 14, 24, 25
Solvents, as irritants, 12, 24
'Soot warts', 136
Spongiosis, 19
Squamous cell carcinoma, 136, 137, 140, 144, 145
Staphylococcal infections, 170
Sticking plaster, 45
Stinging nettles, 108
Stonemasons, 80
Streptococcal infections, 170
'Strimmer rash', 112
Strimmer's phytophotodermatitis, 58, 59, 112
Sunburn, 54, 55
Sunlight, occupational disorders, 53–62
skin cancer, 140–141
see also Ultraviolet light
Swimmer's itch (cercarial dermatitis), 180
Syphilis, 173
Systemic sclerosis, *see* Scleroderma

T
Tar
keratoses, 139, 141
skin cancer, 137, 139
warts, 141
Tattooing, 80
TCDD (2,3,7,8-tetra-chlorodibenzo-*p*-dioxin), 124, 125
T-cells (T-lymphocytes), 32
p-Tertiary butylcatechol, 149, 151, 152, 153
p-Tertiary butylphenol, 149, 150–151
Textile dermatitis, 69
Thioglycolates, 50
Thiourea, 75, 100
Thiuram allergy, 70, 86
Tinea, 177
Trans-epidermal water loss (TEWL), 21
Trees, hardwood, 118–119

Trichophyton species, 177, 178
Trisodium phosphate, 77
Tropical acne, 130, 134
Tuliposide A, 114
Tyrosine, 154, 155

U
UK surveillance reporting scheme (EPI-DERM), 3
Ulcerations, skin, 12, 13
Ultraviolet light, 135
abnormal reactions, 60–62, 110
acute/chronic effects, 54
exposures and sources, 56
normal reactions, 54–56
skin cancer, 140–141
Urticaria, 78
at-risk occupations, 3
cold, 78
contact, 34
delayed pressure, 78
plants and wood causing, 108–109
solar, 61
wheal, 172

V
Vegetables
phototoxic reactions due to, 112
prick test, 108, 109
Vesiculation, 19
Veterinarians, 34, 35, 178
Vibration white finger, 167–168
Vinyl chloride disease, 160
Violinist, 71, 133
Viral infections, 174–176
Vitiligo
idiopathic, 148, 151
occupational, *see* Leukoderma

W
Warts, viral, 102, 176
Water, as irritant, 15, 22, 84
Wax pressmen, 138
Wear and tear dermatitis, 84–85
'Weed wackers' dermatitis', 112
Whitlow, herpetic, 174
Wood dust, 118
Wood, occupational dermatitis, 103–119
allergenic hardwoods, 118
prevention, 119
Wool sorters, 170
Workplace, contact dermatitis prevention, 28
Workplace visits, 10
Work-related health problems, 3

X
Xeroderma pigmentosum, 140
Xerosis, 21
X-ray, *see* Radiograph